Sugar Intake - Risks and Benefits and the Global Diabetes Epidemic

Edited by Ian James Martins

Published in London, United Kingdom

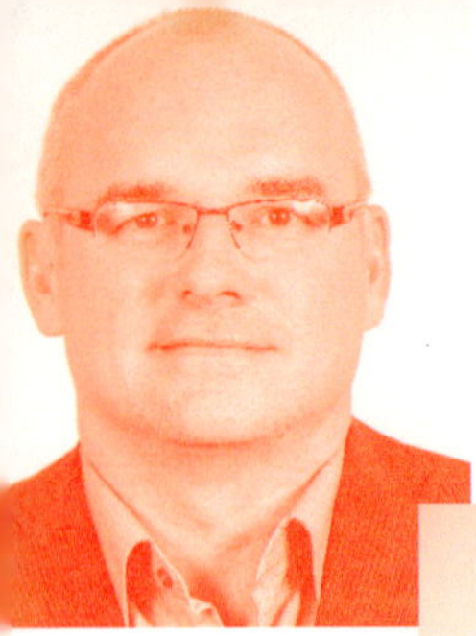
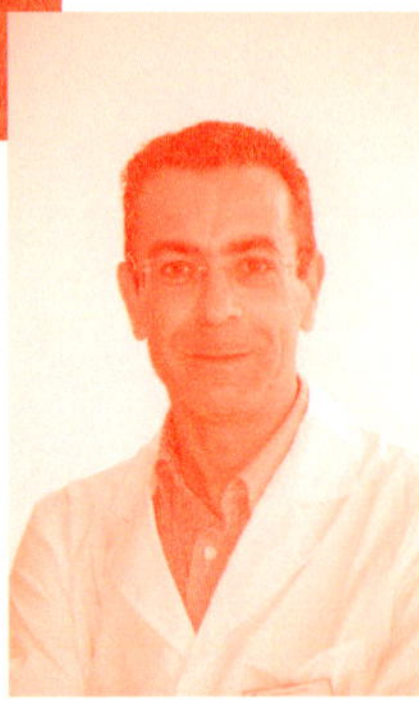
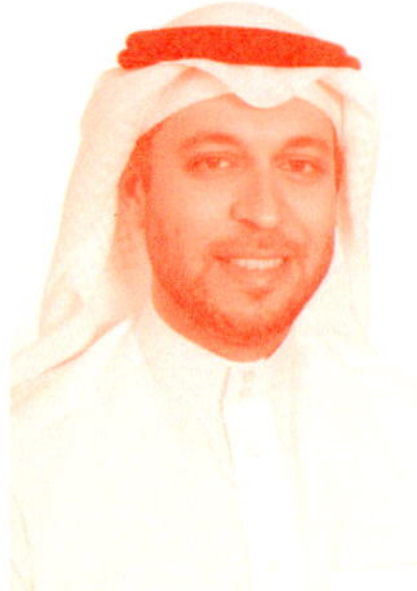
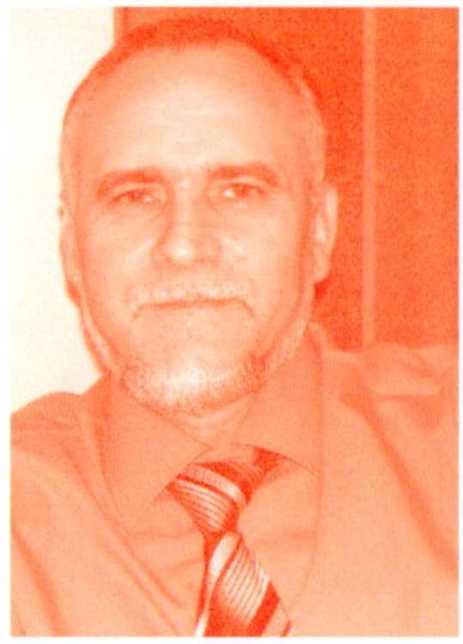
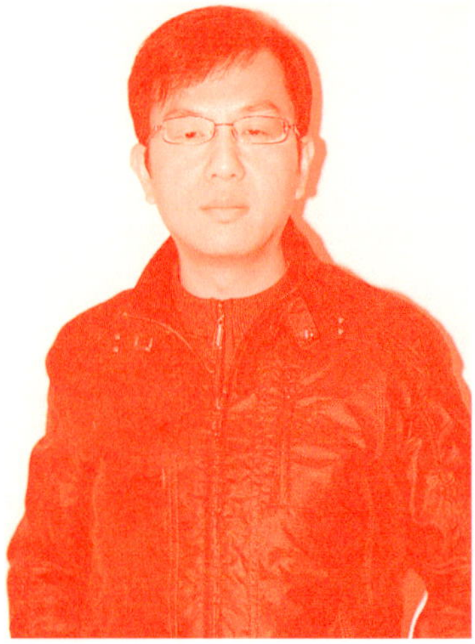
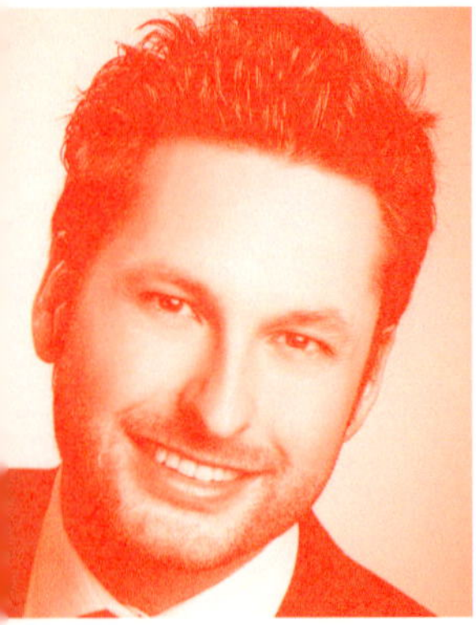
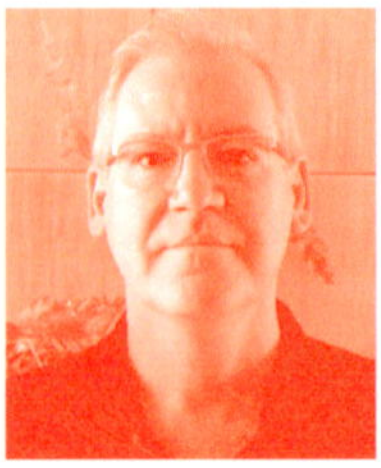

IntechOpen

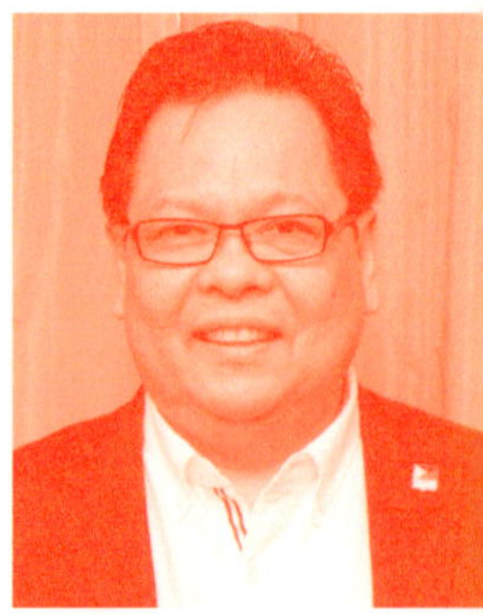
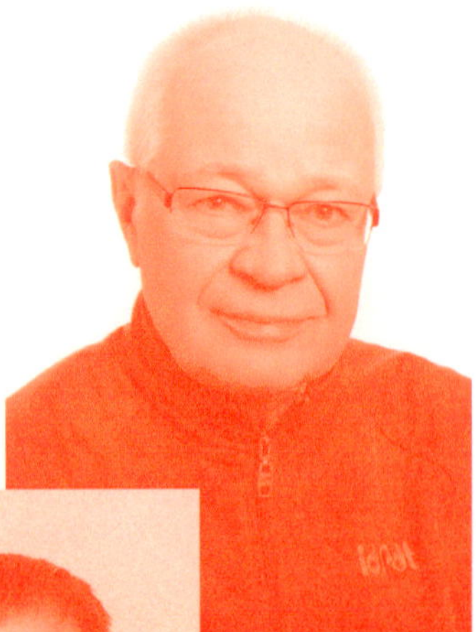
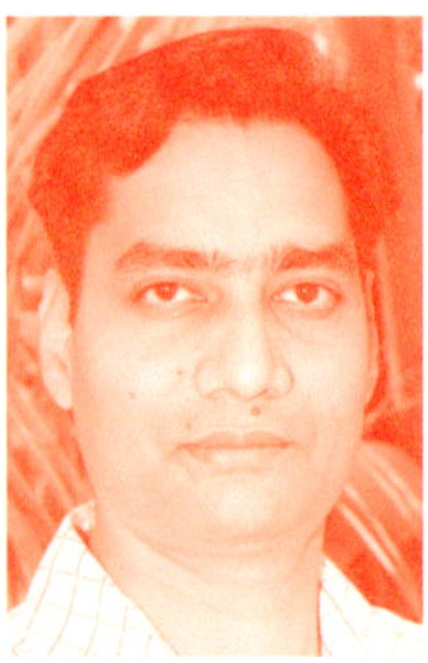
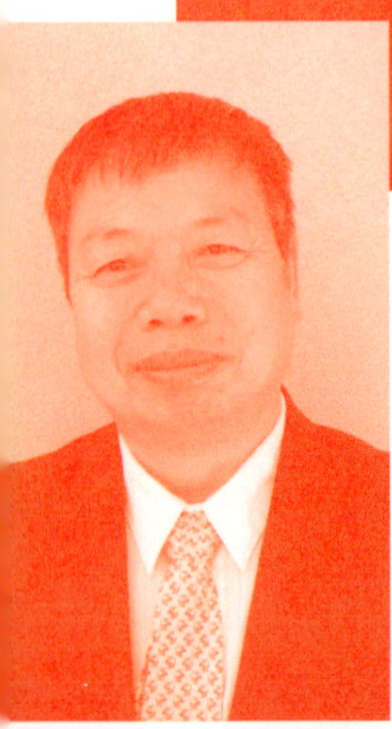
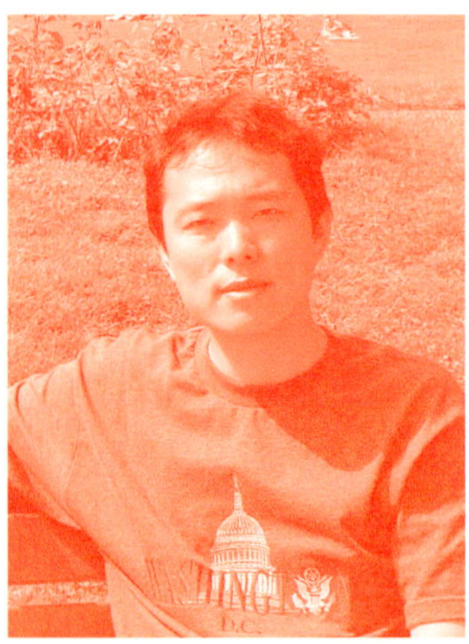
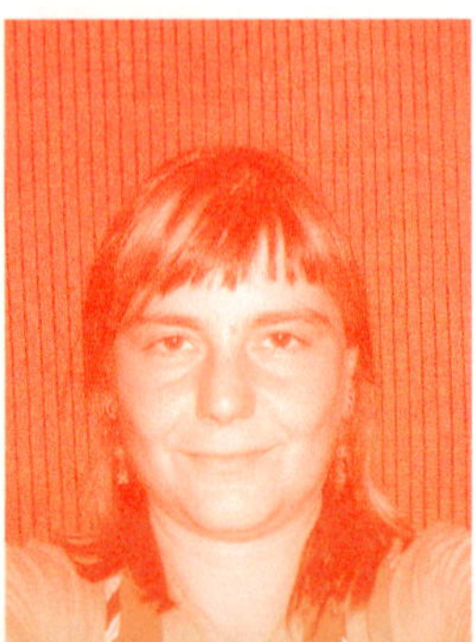

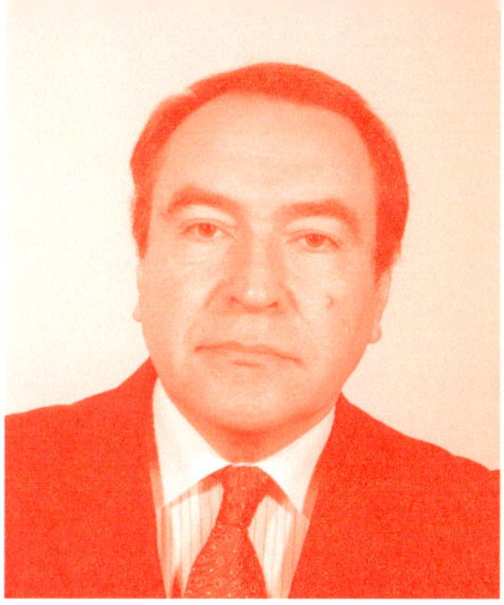
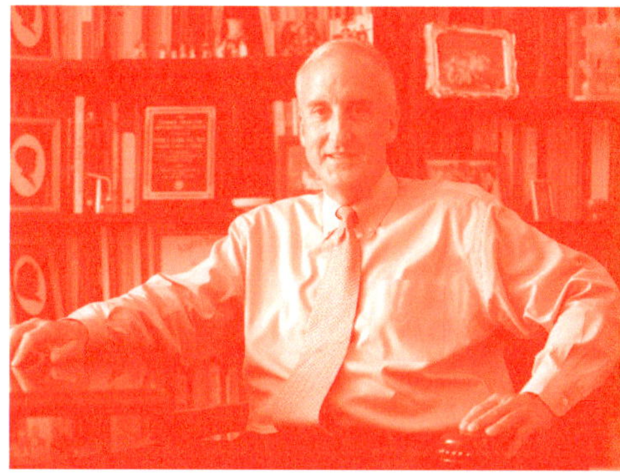
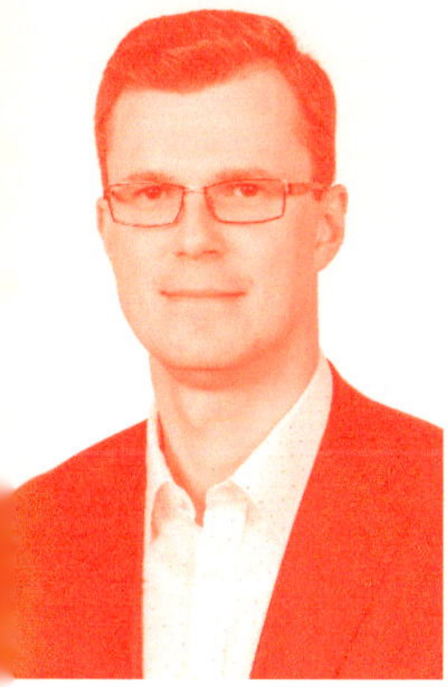
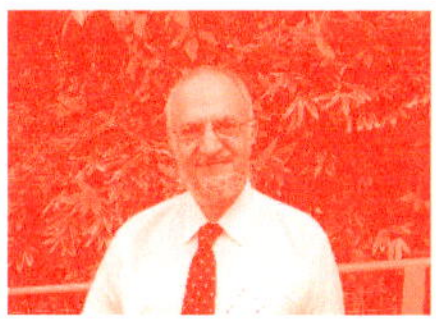
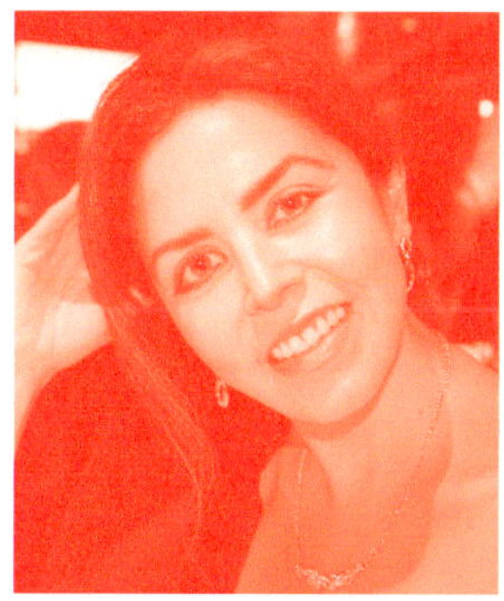

Supporting open minds since 2005

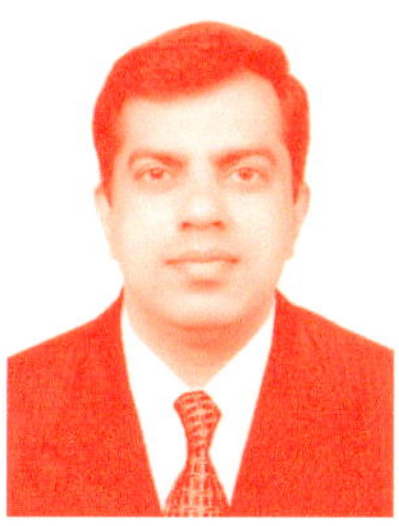
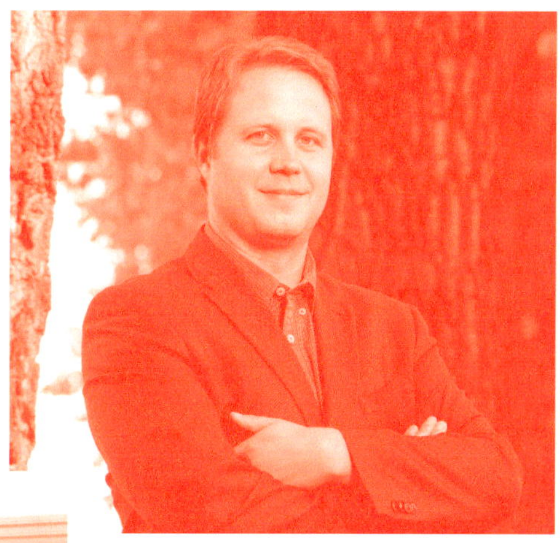
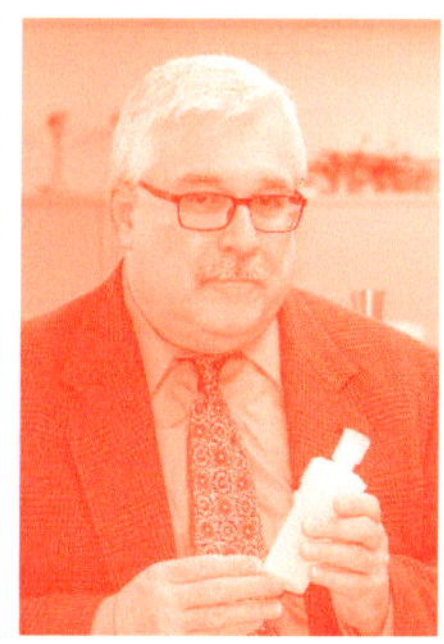
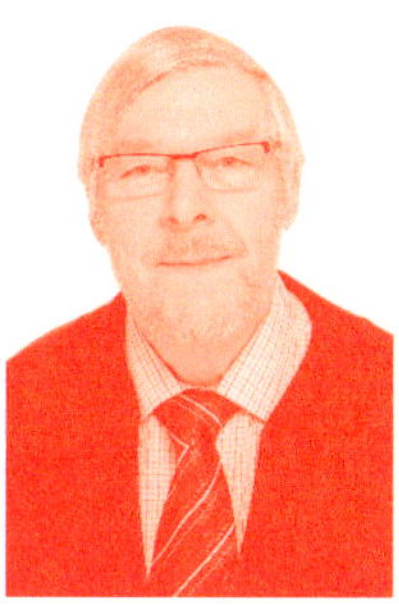
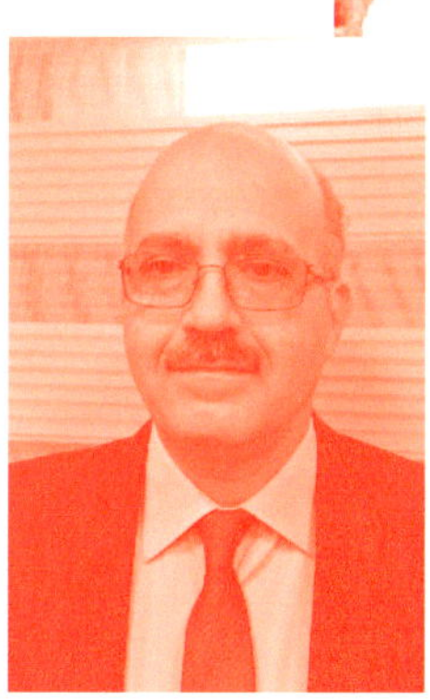
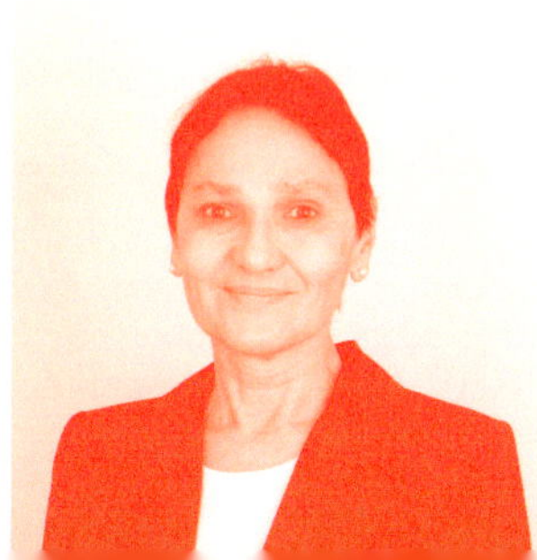
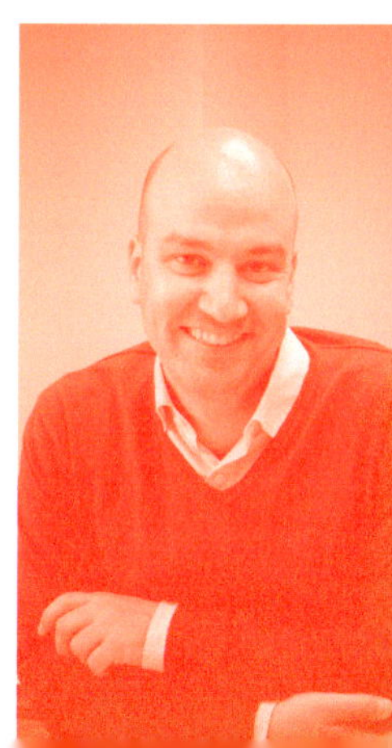

Sugar Intake - Risks and Benefits and the Global Diabetes Epidemic
http://dx.doi.org/10.5772/intechopen.87269
Edited by Ian James Martins

Contributors
Sage Arbor, Tomoya Shintani, Laura Lema-Perez, Hideya Shintani, Koichiro Takagi, Mariko Ueno, Mitsue Muraoka, Frankie B. Stentz, Grace Ogbonna, Rosemary Ehigbo, Hannah Ogbonna, Yun Yan, Wayne V. Moore, Luke He, Ghufran S. Babar, Jacob M. Redel, Sabetha L. Young, Callie Chagas, Kang Li, Ian James Martins

First published in London, United Kingdom, 2021 by IntechOpen
IntechOpen is the global imprint of INTECHOPEN LIMITED, registered in England and Wales, registration number: 11086078, 5 Princes Gate Court, London, SW7 2QJ, United Kingdom
Printed in Croatia

British Library Cataloguing-in-Publication Data
A catalogue record for this book is available from the British Library

Additional hard and PDF copies can be obtained from orders@intechopen.com

Sugar Intake - Risks and Benefits and the Global Diabetes Epidemic
Edited by Ian James Martins
p. cm.
Print ISBN 978-1-83881-121-1
Online ISBN 978-1-83881-122-8
eBook (PDF) ISBN 978-1-83881-167-9

For EU product safety concerns:
IN TECH d.o.o., Prolaz Marije Krucifikse Kozulić 3, 51000 Rijeka, Croatia, info@intechopen.com or visit our website at intechopen.com.

Meet the editor

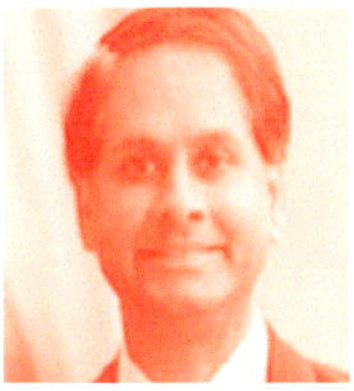

Dr. Ian James Martins has a DSc in Science in Nutrition and an MD in Diabetology. He is an editor and reviewer for various national and international journals. He received the Distinguished Scientist award from the International Scientist Awards on Engineering, Science and Medicine in 2021. He was also recognized as Top Peer Reviewer by the Global Peer Review Awards in 2019. Dr. Martins ranks in the top 1% of cited researchers according to the Essential Science Indicators (ESI) tool. He has an h index of 132 with more than 15,000 citations over the past 27 years. He also has 205 international certificates from journals, conferences, congresses, and summits. Dr. Martins is a member of the BIT Congress.

Contents

Preface

The increase in diabetes cases worldwide is associated with accelerated aging, pancreatic dysfunction, and the induction of various chronic diseases. There is now a type 3 diabetes, which is associated with various brain diseases such as stroke, dementia, and Alzheimer's disease. Sugar intake is critical to healthy aging and determines mitochondrial survival in the pancreas and brain. There is an increased risk for the development of diabetes in both the developing and developed world. Insulin therapy and sugar intake are closely connected to non-alcoholic fatty liver disease (NAFLD) with insulin therapy inactivation associated with brain diseases and NAFLD, which are now major global organ diseases. The recalculation of daily sugar intake is critical to maintain anti-aging genes and to reverse accelerated aging, NAFLD, and neurodegeneration connected to the global diabetes epidemic. Discoveries in genomic medicine and nutrition sciences have become important to maintain insulin dosing and timing in diabetic individuals to prevent the natural progression of hyperglycemia-induced severity of diabetic complications. Medical devices that promote diabetes technology assist with continuous infusion of subcutaneous insulin, which plays an important role in the treatment of diabetes. Preventing micro and macrovascular consequences of prolonged hyperglycemia and delaying the progressive loss of β-cell function are the key goals of anti-diabetes therapies. Key milestones in diabetes technology include the development of the artificial pancreas, which may be one of the most promising treatments ever for this disease. The severity of the global chronic disease epidemic may involve uncontrolled progression that may override basic insulin therapy with costs expected to reach $250 billion dollars. In the United States, unexpected health costs of diabetes are estimated to reach $344 billion dollars by 2040. The use of various anti-hyperglycemic drugs is important to the treatment of diabetes with effects on β-cell function. Major efforts have been made to identify biomarkers of insulin resistance and to delay multiple organ disease syndrome associated with diabetes. The major concern of uncontrolled hyperglycemia and mitochondrial apoptosis in diabetics is the impetus for the publication of this book. Written by experts from around the globe, this book examines the risks and benefits of sugar intake and the critical role of functional foods in treating diabetes. The chapters provide information to control sugar intake and to prevent the induction of organ disease in diabetic individuals. Food restriction and low-calorie diets are critical to reverse multiple organ disease in diabetes and prevent mitochondrial apoptosis, which leads to programmed cell death.

Dr. Ian James Martins
Independent Scientist,
Perth, Australia

References

[1] Martins IJ. Increased Risk for Obesity and Diabetes with Neurodegeneration in Developing Countries. Top 10 Contribution on Genetics. Chapter 1, EBook. 2018. www.avid.science.com

[2] Martins IJ. Functional Foods and Active molecules with relevance to Health and Chronic disease:. Functional Foods in Health and Disease 2017; 7(10): 833-836.

[3] Insulin Therapy Inactivation is connected to NAFLD and Diabetes Severity Index. J Diab Clin Stud. 2017; 1: 001-003.

[4] Martins IJ. Diet and Nutrition reverse Type 3 Diabetes and Accelerated Aging linked to Global chronic diseases. J Diab Res Ther. 2016; 2(2).

[5] Martins IJ. Anti-Aging Genes Improve Appetite Regulation and Reverse Cell Senescence and Apoptosis in Global Populations. Advances in Aging Research, 2016, 5, 9-26

[6] Martins IJ. Diabetes and Organ Dysfunction in the Developing and Developed. World Global Journal of Medical Research: F Diseases Volume 15 Issue 1 Version 1.0 Year 2015.

[7] Martins IJ. Insulin Therapy and Autoimmune Disease with Relevance to Nonalcoholic Fatty Liver Disease. Non Alcoholic Fatty Liver Disease. An Update. IntechOpen. 2018.

Chapter 1

Introductory Chapter: Sugar Intake and Global Chronic Disease

Ian James Martins

1. Introduction

The incidence of diabetes has been predicted to increase to 21% by 2050. In various continents, the rise in the global diabetes epidemic has been associated with diseases of various organs related to obesity, diabetes and neurodegenerative diseases [1]. Type 2 diabetes is now connected to Type 3 diabetes that involves the brain early in life associated with various brain diseases such as stroke, dementia, and Alzheimer's disease. Sugar intake is now critical to healthy aging and determines mitochondrial survival [2] and the lifespan of diabetics in the developing and developed world (**Figure 1**). The risk of sugar (glucose, fructose) intake is associated with amyloid-beta aggregation and programmed cell death relevant to neurodegeneration and Alzheimer's disease. Insulin therapy and sugar intake are closely connected to the global non-alcoholic fatty liver disease (NAFLD) with insulin therapy inactivation associated with the induction of NAFLD [1]. Food quality [3] is critical to the global diabetes epidemic with recalculation of daily sugar intake essential to maintain the anti-aging gene and to reverse accelerated aging, NAFLD and neurodegeneration.

The guidelines on dietary sugar require critical recommendations [4] with relevance to functional food science. Food scientists indicate that functional foods contain biologically active compounds that have advantageous physiological effects that play an important role in the prevention of insulin resistance. Nutritional science provides functional foods with the required amounts of natural compounds [5] that prevent mitophagy and reverse programmed cell death. This book contains chapters that assist food scientists with relevance to sugar intake (risks and benefits) and are

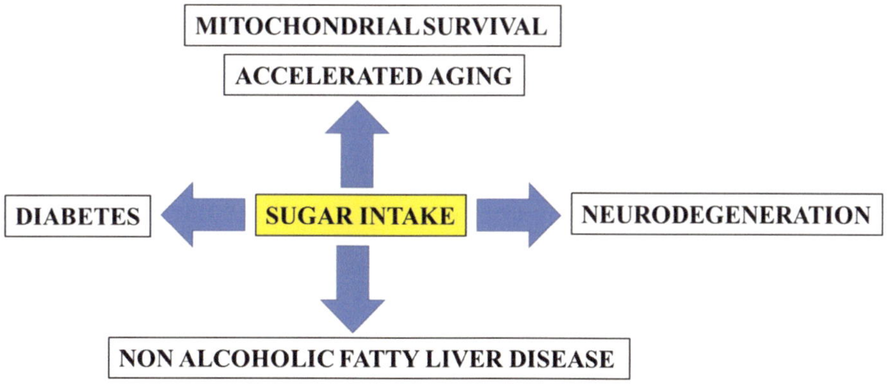

Figure 1.
The role of sugar intake is critical to mitochondrial survival that is connected to diabetes, NAFLD and Alzheimer's disease.

important to the critical role played by functional foods in the treatment of individuals from the global chronic disease. The chapters published in this book are from various authors around the world. These authors have written excellent chapters that maintain the high standards for the best book companies. The quality of the research contributed in chapters include research on the impact of sugar on vision, use of pedometer for the management of impaired glucose intolerance, fructose intake with relevance to metabolism and severity in chronic diseases. The role of organs involved in glucose metabolism and the effect of ad framing on the intention to control sugar intake is assessed. The biological responses to the consumption of non-nutritional sweeteners is assessed with the role of hyperglycemia and hyperlipidemia induced activation of human T lymphocytes and inflammation and inhibition by ω- 3 Fatty Acid. The research on critical elements of dietary carbohydrates and the metabolic syndrome with relevance to the sugars with the potential to prolong human life are discussed in this scholarly book. The research contributed in these chapters by the authors is of key interest to functional foods and the current global chronic disease epidemic. The role of anti-aging genes [6, 7] are of critical interest that when activated will reverse impaired glucose tolerance, improve vision, extend life and improve the metabolic syndrome in diabetes. The research mentioned in these chapters will improve the anti-aging gene release of anti-aging proteins [8] that are critical to longevity and reversal of the global chronic disease epidemic. The risk and benefits of sugar intake as outlined in this book may revolve around the activation and repression of the anti-aging gene that is critical to mitochondrial survival and if the question with relevance to risks and benefits of sugar intake remains unanswered it may lead to the predicted global increase in NAFLD, diabetes and neurodegenerative disease by the year 2050.

Author details

Ian James Martins
Independent Scientist, Australia

*Address all correspondence to: fellow.iasr@gmail.com; i.martins@ecu.edu.au

References

[1] Martins IJ. Insulin Therapy and Autoimmune Disease with Relevance to Nonalcoholic Fatty Liver Disease. Non Alcoholic Fatty Liver Disease. An Update. IntechOpen. 2018.

[2] Martins IJ. Increased Risk for Obesity and Diabetes with Neurodegeneration in Developing Countries. Top 10 Contribution on Genetics. Chapter 1, EBook. 2018. www.avid.science.com

[3] Martins, IJ. Overnutrition determines LPS regulation of mycotoxin induced neurotoxicity in neurodegenerative diseases. Int J Mol Sci. 2015; 16(12): 29554-29573.

[4] Erickson J, Sadeghirad B, Lytvyn L, Slavin J, Johnston BC. The scientific basis of guideline recommendations on sugar intake: A systematic review. Ann Intern Med. 2017;166(4):257-267.

[5] Martins IJ. Functional foods and active molecules with relevance to health and chronic disease: Editorial. Functional Foods in Health and Disease 2017; 7(10): 833-836.

[6] Martins, IJ. Anti-aging genes improve appetite regulation and reverse cell senescence and apoptosis in global populations. Advances in Aging Research, 2016, 5, 9-26.

[7] Martins, IJ. Single gene inactivation with implications to diabetes and multiple organ dysfunction syndrome. J Clin Epigenet. 2017; Vol. 3 No. 3:24.

[8] Martins, IJ. Sirtuin 1, a diagnostic protein marker and its relevance to chronic disease and therapeutic drug interventions". EC Pharmacology and Toxicology 6.4 (2018): 209-215.

Chapter 2

The Sugars with the Potential to Prolong Human Life

Tomoya Shintani, Laura Lema-Perez and Hideya Shintani

Abstract

Sugar is the main source of energy for all cells in the human body. On the other hand, cells can also obtain energy from fats and proteins depending on conditions, although this metabolic process is more difficult and less common in cells. Sugar intake has increased in recent decades and is included in most of our dietary products. However, many studies indicate that sugar intake increases the prevalence of suffering from various harmful health conditions such as obesity. As a consequence, obesity is related to several chronic diseases such as hypertension, insulin resistance, and diabetes mellitus in humans. This is due to an excessive intake of sugars and sedentary lifestyles, causing a deterioration in the organs of our body, and consequently, reducing life expectancy. In this chapter, sugars that both shorten and lengthen life expectancy are presented. The latter are recent options that have emerged in order to continue sweetening our food in a healthier way, and would be new geroprotectors.

Keywords: Lifespan, healthy life, sugar, glucose metabolism

1. Introduction

Sugar is the main source of energy for the cells of the human body and is a nutrient that is abundantly found in nature and is widely used in the food processing industry. In the 1970s and 1980s, a strong association was found between cardiovascular disease, the number 1 cause of death in the world, and fat intake. For this reason, the food industry began to create low-fat but high-sugar consumer products. Today there is evidence that the high consumption of sugars in the recent decades has triggered a lot of chronic diseases that were not previously known, as diabetes mellitus. The appearance of chronic diseases such as diabetes mellitus has increased exponentially. Diabetes mellitus, e.g., is considered today a pandemic, due to it is one of the most prevalent not transmissible diseases in the world. The role sugar intake that is linked to aging is now relevant to the global chronic disease epidemic [1]. The global nonalcoholic fatty liver disease epidemic also has now become of major concern to diabetes [2].

Many scientific studies show that the increase in chronic diseases is due to excessive consumption of sugars and low-quality carbohydrates. This chapter presents in Section 2 the relationship between human life expectancy and sugar consumption, including a brief explanation of glucose metabolism in the human body. Later, Section 3 presents sugars as glucose, fructose, and galactose known as likely to shorten life with excessive intake. On the other hand, Section 4 presents sugar with potential to extend life expectancy like 2-deoxy-glucose, allulose, and glucosamine. Finally, the conclusions are presented.

2. Interaction of lifespan and sugar

2.1 Sugar consumption in human

Humans are always aging. The progress of aging and the life span are affected by environmental factors inside and outside the living body. One of the most promising environmental factors is oxidative stress. The free radical theory of aging is based on the idea that active oxygen, which is a causative agent of oxidative stress, oxidatively damages biomolecules and causes their accumulation to cause a decline in cell function, which causes aging [3]. Active oxygen is considered as a cause of various diseases as well as aging. Therefore, "antioxidant therapy" has been devised, which aims to treat diseases by controlling active oxygen as a toxic factor.

The generation of active oxygen is largely related to mitochondria. The main physiological role of mitochondria is to produce energy, or ATP. The ATP synthetic pathway includes anaerobic glycolysis that does not require oxygen and aerobic oxidative phosphorylation that requires oxygen [4]. The primary function of mitochondria is this oxidative phosphorylation. That is, by utilizing oxygen, more ATP is produced more efficiently than the glycolytic system. This oxidative phosphorylation is carried out by the electron transfer system existing in the inner mitochondrial membrane. About 100 kinds of proteins are involved in the electron transfer system, and various enzymes form a complex (Complex I to IV). In mitochondria, surprisingly, in addition to oxidative phosphorylation, metabolism such as ion channels, intracellular calcium homeostasis, fatty acid β-oxidation, neutral fat cycle, urea cycle, amino, fat, heme, purine, steroid and steroid hormone synthesis. It has various functions related to. Normally, 2 to 3% of electrons leak from the electron transport system, and the leaked electrons react with the most reactive oxygen molecule in the vicinity to produce superoxide.

Active oxygen is generated not only by external factors but also by internal factors. In mitochondria, active oxygen is produced as a by-product during the process of energy production. Some phagocytic cells produce active oxygen for the treatment of foreign substances such as bacteria. In some aspects, active oxygen is not necessarily an unfavorable existence for living things. Subsequent studies have revealed that active oxygen has a role as a physiologically active substance and a redox signal molecule [5, 6].

2.2 ROS generation and mitochondrial respiration

Complex I and Complex III are well known as the main generation sites of superoxide [7, 8]. Complex II also contributes to active oxygen produced from mitochondria [9]. Other mitochondrial enzymes that are not directly involved in the electron transport system also play a part in the production of mitochondrial active oxygen, and dihydroorotic acid oxidase is a by-product during the conversion of dihydroorotic acid to orotic acid and also the TCA (tricarboxylic acid) cycle. It has been reported that α-ketoglutarate dehydrogenase, which is an enzyme of *Escherichia coli*, also produces NADH/NAD+-dependent active oxygen [10, 11].

The mitochondrial oxidative metabolism of glucose is the most commonly known mechanism through which the ingestion of carbohydrates generates oxidative stress. Mitochondrial oxidative metabolism of glucose leads to the generation of reactive oxygen species (ROS). When glucose intake is high, glucose levels in the bloodstream rise, increasing many metabolic processes inside the cells regarding glucose metabolism, consequently increasing the ROS, and including the auto-oxidation, through the mitochondria. The mitochondrial respiration chain generates free radicals as a result of electron transport and depletion of the oxygen molecule.

Higher glucose consumption in the cell from the mitochondria causes a higher number of ROS [12]. Several studies [13] indicate that ROS, extremely reactive chemical molecules, are the major cause of the aging process in humans.

2.3 Hormesis

Hormesis is a biphasic response to exposure to increasing amounts of a substance [14]. Within the hormesis, there is generally a relatively favorable biological response to low exposures to toxic substances and other stressors. The concept of hormesis has been explored extensively with respect to its applicability is aging [15]. Because the survival capacity of any biological system is dependent on its defensive ability, exposing organisms to stress is expected to result in the adaptive response with various benefits. This idea has now gathered a large body of supportive evidence showing that repetitive mild stress exposure has anti-aging effects [16, 17]. Hormetic interventions have also been proposed at the clinical level [18], with a variety of stimuli, challenges and stressful actions, that aim to increase the dynamical complexity of the biological systems in humans [19].

ROS, which mentioned above, may perform an important lifespan-depending role as redox signaling molecules which transduce signals from the mitochondrial compartment to other compartments of the cell [20]. Increased temporarily formation of ROS within the mitochondria may cause an hormesis effect and reaction which induces increased stress resistance and a long-term reduction of oxidative stress. This type of reverse effect of the response to ROS stress has been named mitochondrial hormesis and is hypothesized to be responsible for the respective lifespan-extending capabilities of glucose restriction [20].

2.4 Sugar metabolism

Life is active. Energy is essential for activities. The most important source of energy for the cells of the human body is glucose. They create energy from glucose to stay alive and to carry out many metabolic processes in different organs and tissues. Humans have easy access to glucose. Glucose enters the human body through the mouth, where it begins to be processed by the amylases contained in saliva [21]. After that, the glucose travels up the esophagus to the stomach. Glucose and carbohydrates in general that reach the stomach do not undergo chemical or mechanical changes, since the enzymes that degrade them are not active at the acid pH that is in the stomach. The glucose then reaches the intestine, where it is absorbed into the bloodstream through the intestinal wall [21]. Then, glucose is metabolized in the liver thanks to the action of insulin. Excess glucose is stored as glycogen, while a quantity of glucose continues into the systemic circulation through the hepatic veins. Thus, glucose reaches all tissues to be used in cellular mitochondria as energy.

Glucose is absorbed quickly, whereas fructose is converted to glucose (10%) and the remaining 90% is absorbed as fructose. Sixty percent of the absorbed glucose is taken up by other tissues, such as the liver, 25% by the brain, 10% by muscle, and 5% by adipose tissue [22]. Meanwhile, almost all of the absorbed fructose is taken up by the liver. The glucose and fructose taken up by the liver is consumed in the glycolytic system, through the TCA cycle, and in ATP production, with the excess converted to glycogen and triglycerides. However, there is a major metabolic difference between glucose and fructose in the liver. Glucose is regulated by the insulin-dependent metabolic rate-limiting enzymes glucokinase, phospho-fructokinase, and glycogen synthase, but in the case of fructose, this regulatory mechanism does not work well. Fructose is mostly phosphorylated by fructokinase. However, there is no mechanism to control the phosphorylation of fructose and its subsequent metabolism. Therefore, the influx of excess fructose into the liver leads to increased synthesis of triglycerides and release of triglycerides into the blood, resulting in hypertriglyceridemia because of the limited glycogen stores in the liver [23]. This process is especially active in diabetes mellitus with insufficient insulin action, because glycogen synthesis and ATP production are not as smooth as they could be.

3. Sugars with the potential to shorten human life

Glucose, fructose, and galactose are sugars that are likely to be short-lived with excessive intake. Specific characteristics of each one of them are presented in this section.

3.1 Glucose

Glucose is a simple sugar with the molecular formula $C_6H_{12}O_6$, as shown in **Figure 1**. Glucose is the most abundant monosaccharide, a subcategory of carbohydrates. Glucose is mainly made by plants and most algae during photosynthesis from water and carbon dioxide, using energy from sunlight, where it is used to make cellulose in cell walls, which is the most abundant carbohydrate [24]. In energy metabolism, glucose is the most important source of energy in all organisms. Glucose for metabolism is stored as a polymer, in plants mainly as starch and amylopectin, and in animals and humans as glycogen. Glucose circulates in the blood of animals as blood sugar. Glucose in the blood is the source of energy for cells throughout the body and is supplied through food intake and transported through the bloodstream.

Excessive glucose intake is directly linked to diabetes. Diabetes mellitus is one of the most prevalent chronic non-communicable diseases today. Type 2 diabetes mellitus (DM) is a progressive disease by uncontrolled plasma glucose levels. In the epidemiological study drawn from the general population, random glucose consumption showed a significant association with all-cause mortality, independent of main potential confounders [25]. Thus, random glucose measures are highly relevant to health risk assessment among people without known diabetes when fasting glucose or HbA1c is difficult to obtain.

DM results from a combination of factors affecting both insulin sensitivity and β-cell function. Chronic hyperglycemia imposes glucose toxicity on many cell types and is correlated with the myriad of DM-related complications [26]. Cells most vulnerable to the effects of prolonged elevated plasma glucose levels include pancreatic cells and vascular endothelial cells. The ensuing pancreatic dysfunction promotes decreased

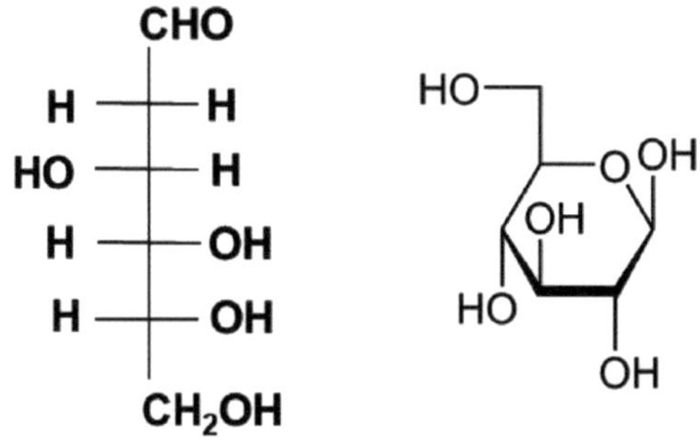

Figure 1.
Linear chemical structure (left) and Haworth projection structure (right) of a glucose molecule.

insulin secretion, further perpetuating the associated hyperglycemia. On the vascular endothelium, chronic hyperglycemia is correlated with some types of DM-related microvascular complications, including retinopathy and nephropathy [26].

3.2 Fructose

Fructose is contained in many fruits, vegetables, and honey. It is a monosaccharide with the same molecular formula as glucose ($C_6H_{12}O_6$), but with a different structure (see **Figure 2**), that is, it is an isomer of it. An increase intake of sugars, including fructose, in beverages is related to high prevalence of having obesity, type 2 DM, insulin resistance, hyperinsulinemia, and hypertension in humans. These chronic diseases without a good treatment or if they are not well controlled, cause a decrease in life expectancy. Nowadays, there is little scientific evidence for the fructose and its relationship with life expectancy in humans. It is known that fructose metabolism mainly occurs in the enterocytes (cells of the small intestine), hepatocytes (cells in the liver), and nephrons (cells in the kidneys) [27]. Nevertheless, few studies indicate that fructose could extend lifespan in some organisms as the nematode, fly and mice. This is due to life of many of those organisms, including yeast, is regulated by the insulin/IGF-1(Insulin-like Growth Factor-1)-signaling pathway [28].

On the other hand, high fructose corn syrup (HFCS) is commercially produced by isomerizing glucose to fructose. The taste quality of it is like sucrose and the price is affordable. This monosaccharide is a component of sucrose and is highly sweet (140% the sweetness of sucrose), leading to its frequent use in the food industry, particularly for beverage production. Thus, fructose consumption is common in the beverage industry, in which more sweetness is often needed [29]. In the field, fructose is used as a mixture of fructose and glucose, e.g., high fructose corn syrup, which is easy and inexpensive to manufacture from glucose. Thus, HFCS has been used for various foods such as beverages, confectionery, desserts and bakery. However, consumption of HFCS has been reported to be one of risk factors developing diabetes and obesity [30]. Sirtuin 1 is an anti-aging gene that becomes downregulated with relevance to the global chronic disease epidemic. Glucose and Fructose induce changes in Sirtuin 1 protein levels with relevance to induction of the metabolic syndrome and multiple organ disease syndrome [31]. Consumption of glucose and fructose should be carefully monitored with relevance to plasma Sirtuin 1 levels that now are connected to obesity, diabetes, NAFLD and neurodegenerative diseases [32]. Fructose induces gluconeogenesis and lipogenesis [33]. Excessive intake of fructose has been reported to result in short life [34].

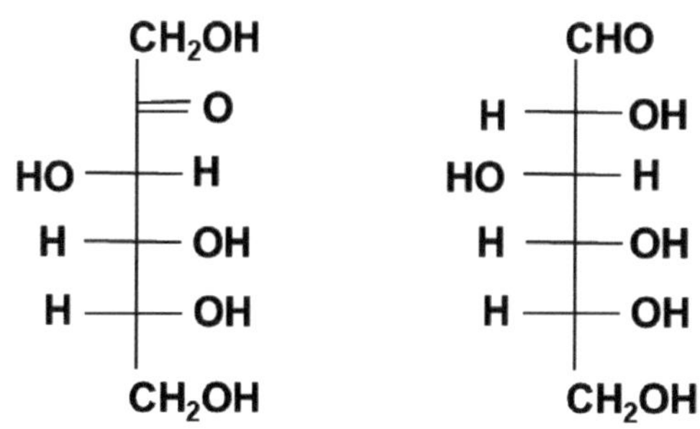

Figure 2.
Linear chemical structures of a fructose molecule (left) and a glucose molecule (right).

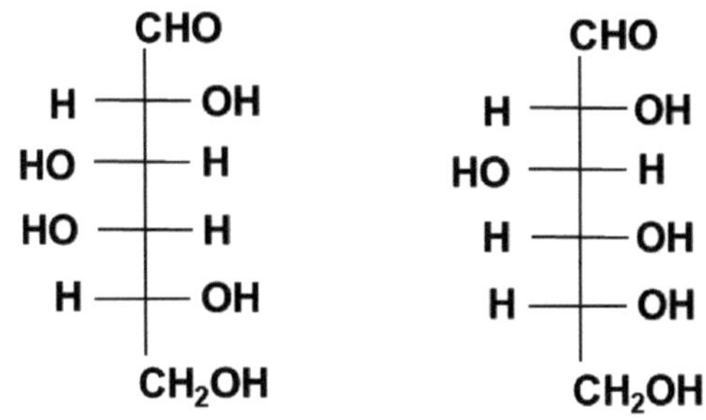

Figure 3.
Linear chemical structures of a galactose molecule (left) and a glucose molecule (right).

3.3 Galactose

Galactose is a C-4 epimer of glucose, as can be seen in **Figure 3**. Galactose, along with fructose and glucose, is an essential simple sugar included in the human diet. Galactose is a component of lactose, the disaccharide of which is contained in approximately 10% of milk. Lactose is a disaccharide that makes up around 3–7% of milk [35] and is derived from the condensation of galactose and glucose, which forms a β-glycosidic bond. Therefore, galactose can be consumed individually or in combination with other sugars in the form of more complex carbohydrates [36] to be digested and absorbed mainly in the small intestine into the bloodstream. In addition to being absorbed through the small intestine, some reports indicate that the human body can produce galactose endogenously [37] under some metabolic disorders associated with genetic mutations in enzymes of the Leloir pathway [38].

Many volumes of the disaccharides are produced annually as a by-product of the dairy industry [39]. Milk is consumed by people worldwide. However, lactose in milk may cause health problems in individuals with lactose intolerance [40, 41]. Thus, methods for lactose degradation in milk have been extensively studied [42, 43] and the lactose-free milk is produced and commercialized. In this case, studies have been conducted to assess blood glucose levels when lactose-free milk is consumed and a tendency to hyperglycemia was found 2 hours after consumption even in healthy people. The condition of hyperglycemia can be caused because lactose is ingested in its simplest forms, galactose, and glucose, and therefore it can be absorbed directly in the small intestine into the bloodstream, without going through digestion processes in the gastrointestinal tract. On the other hand, galactose can be produced industrially by lactase (β-galactosidase) derived from food microorganisms [44]. However, due to its low sweetness and limited research regarding its safety and functions [45], utilization of pure galactose in the food industry is not yet widespread [46]. Many animal studies have showed galactose induced accelerated aging in rodents [47, 48].

4. Sugars with the potential to prolong human life

2-Deoxy-glucose (2DG), allulose (AL), and glucosamine (GN) are sugars that are likely to be prolong life with intake. These monosaccharides would be new geroprotectors. This section describes a brief detail of all of them.

4.1 2-Deoxy-glucose

2DG is a glucose analog in which the 2-hydroxyl group is replaced by a hydrogen atom, as shown in **Figure 4**. 2DG is not at all metabolized via glycolysis and was

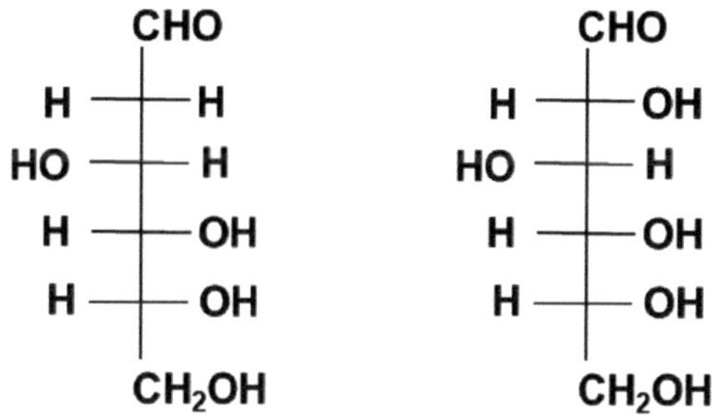

Figure 4.
Linear chemical structures of a 2-deoxy-glucose molecule (left) and a glucose molecule (right).

the first proposed calorie restriction mimetic [49]. It is considered to delay aging-related diseases and prolong the lifespan by suppressing glycolytic activity [50]. Schulz et al. [51] suggested a detailed mechanism for the 2DG longevity effect in *C. elegans* based on a hypothesis named as "mitochondrial hormesis". The hypothesis means that induction of mitochondrial metabolism may trigger a positive response to increased formation of ROS, leading to a hermetic increase in defense for stresses, resulting in decreased total stress levels. Inhibition of glycolysis by 2DG induces the utilization of stored lipid and mitochondrial respiration via AMPK (AMP-activated protein kinase). In a study comparing the effects of 2DG and calorie restriction in rodents, 2DG administration showed the same effects on locomotory activity, heart rate, and blood pressure as calorie restriction [52].

The same group of rodents demonstrated the protective effect of 2DG against glutamate excitotoxicity and upregulation of stress response proteins, in hippocampal cells [53]. Moreover, the same group demonstrated an improved behavioral outcome of 2DG treatment and reduced degeneration of dopaminergic neurons in a Parkinson's disease model [54], as well as decreases in proliferating cell nuclear antigen and bromodeoxyuridine-positive tumor cells [55]. On the other hand, a study in nematodes [56] found that the magnitude of gene expression values changes significantly when they are feeding with 2DG, the change is proportional to the age, but the most important thing is that their lifespan could be considerably extended.

Although 2DG shows the same effects as calorie restriction, few studies have examined its ability to extend lifespan. Rather, long-term 2DG ingestion induced heart vacuolation in rats and increased mortality [57]. However, 2DG is considered a potential caloric restriction mimetic due to it has effects on the metabolism that might regulate increases of the stress responses which protect against several aging processes, by improving longevity without a reduction or complete suppression of food intake. In this sense, Ingram et al. [58] shown that the use of 2DG reduces body temperatures, Dark et al. [59] report an increment of lethargy, Wan et al. [60] support a reduction of heart rate, and other studies indicate a declination of insulin and glucose blood levels [61, 62].

4.2 Allulose

Allulose (AL; psicose), a C-3 epimer of fructose (see **Figure 5**), is a rare hexose sugar present in a limited quantity in nature. In fact, this compound is isolated from natural products marketed as a functional sweetener with zero calories [62], easy to produce from d-fructose, in order to use it as a healthier sweetener in industrialized products.

In the previous decade, numerous studies showed that AL exhibits various activities, such as antihyperglycemic and antiobesity effects [63, 64], increment in the insulin sensitivity, attenuate cognitive impairment, delay diseases of aging,

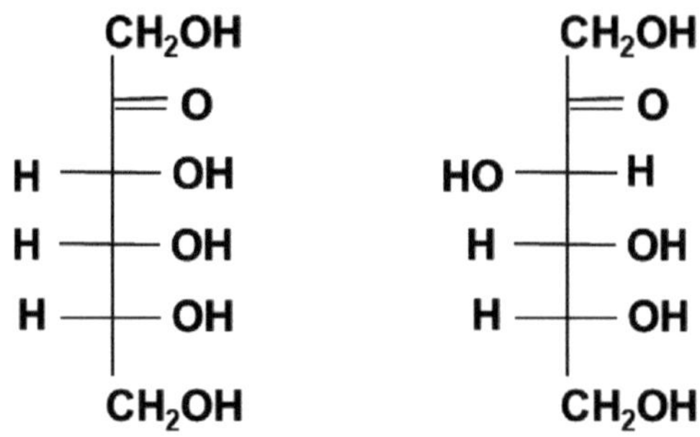

Figure 5.
Linear chemical structures of an allulose molecule (left) and a fructose molecule (right).

slow down cardiac aging, and prolong median life span [65, 66]. Toyoda et al. [67] reported that long-term administration of AL maintained glucose tolerance and insulin sensitivity in rats via hepatic glucokinase activation. Thus, AL is expected to be a potent antidiabetic sweetener. AL enters cells through glucose transporters and inhibits glycolysis, inducing the metabolism of stored fat and mitochondrial respiration via AMPK. Increased respiration causes temporary upregulation of ROS production, leading to increased antioxidant activity, oxidative stress resistance, and survival rates [68]. Although sirtuin is reported to be antiaging gene and a diagnostic marker to chronic disease [31], AL-mediated lifespan extension is independent of sirtuin gene.

In a clinical trial, AL was shown to be a geroprotector based on changes in biomarker levels such as glucose and body fat. A clinical trial using a standard meal confirmed that AL suppresses postprandial blood glucose levels [69]. Even a single dose of AL was reported to enhance postprandial fat oxidation in healthy humans [70]. Upon continuous intake of AL, the percentage of body fat and body fat mass significantly decreased, with no significant reduction in nutrient intake [71].

4.3 Glucosamine

GlcN is, a one of glucose derivatives, 2-amino-2-deoxy-glucose, as can be seen in **Figure 6**. GlcN is part of the structure of two polysaccharides, chitosan and chitin. GlcN is the fluid that surrounds the joints, but also is a constitutional unit of chitosan, which are contained in arthropods and cephalopods. In food industry, GlcN is manufactured by the hydrolysis of crustacean exoskeletons, which are mainly composed of chitin. GlcN is a dietary supplement that effectively prevents osteoarthritis in humans [72].

Weimer et al. reported the longevity effects of GlcN in nematodes and genetically modified mice [73]. The authors suggested that these effects were caused by impaired glucose metabolism. In contrast, the longevity effect of GlcN is reported to be required an autophagy for GlcN-induced lifespan extension [68], like that induced by other life-promoting sugars such as 2DG. Similar to 2DG, GlcN enters into cells through sugar transporters and inhibits glucose metabolism, inducing the oxidation of stored fat and intracellular respiration via an energy sensor (AMPK). Increased respiration can cause temporary production of ROS, leading to increases in antioxidative enzyme activity, stress resistance, and lifespan [74]. This effect is hormesis, mentioned above. Oral administration of GlcN has also been reported to affect carbohydrate metabolism and reduce fat in rodents [75] and contribute to enhanced oxidative stress resistance, followed by AMPK activation [74].

In a clinical trial, administration of GlcN improved vascular endothelial function by modulating the intracellular redox state [76]. According to an

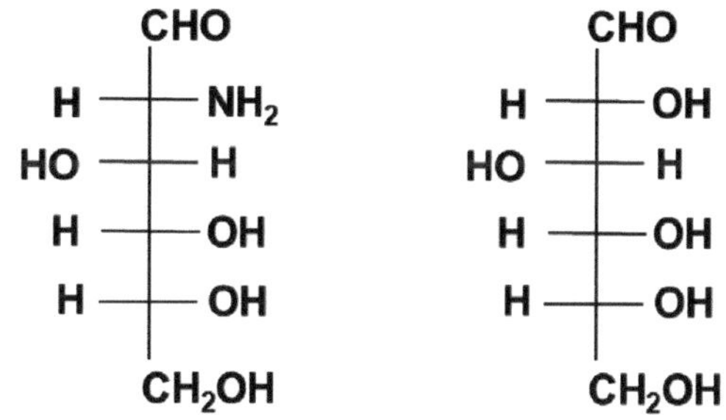

Figure 6.
Linear chemical structures of a glucosamine molecule (left) and a glucose molecule (right).

epidemiological study on consumers of various dietary supplements, the use of GlcN was associated with a decrease in total mortality [77]. Of further note is the latest large-scale cohort study reported in 2020. This study analyzed approximately 500,000 people and found that GlcN intake reduced the risk of cancer, heart disease, respiratory disease, digestive disease, and mortality [78].

5. Geroprotectors

"Geroprotector", whose technical term Ilya Mechnikov first used in 1908 [79], means "protecting against aging". The most important criterion of geroprotector is the ability to extend the lifespan of model organisms such as nematode fly and mice [80]. In 2001, Vladimir Anisimov suggested several types of geroprotectors using the most recognized theories of aging at that time as the typing criteria, which included antioxidants, neurotropic substances, hormones, antidiabetic drugs, immunomodulators, caloric restriction mimetics, and other substances and factors [81]. In the present, the various types would add longevity gene activators, including nicotinamide mononucleotide [82] and sirtuin activating compounds [83], as a new group to these conventional geroprotectors. Other new geroprotectors contain melatonin [84], and carnosine [85]. Among geroprotectors, the monosaccharides with the potential to prolong lifespan, mentioned in this chapter, is included in category of caloric restriction mimetics [49, 50]. This type of caloric restriction mimetics, whose action is considered glycolytic inhibition, mimics the anti-aging effects of long-term calorie restriction without requiring a change in eating habits [68].

6. Conclusion

Sugar consumption has increased since the 1990s when scientific studies found a strong association between fat consumption and cardiovascular problems. Since then, fats were almost sensed and sugars and carbohydrates were given priority. Sugar consumption has increased so much that it has triggered an enormous number of chronic diseases such as obesity and diabetes mellitus that, even today, have been declared a pandemic and a global emergency. Diseases caused by high sugar consumption generate a decline in the organs of the human body, which is closely linked to premature aging or a significant reduction in the quality of life of the people who suffer from them. In this regard, many studies have evidence that sugar intake to have effects in the human body associated with diseases as obesity and diabetes mellitus, however, little was until recently known about the effects of sugars on lifespan. As mentioned in this chapter, sugars that both shorten and lengthen life expectancy was presented. The good options with antiaging effect of the sugars have emerged in order to continue sweetening our food in a healthier way. It would be new geroprotectors in the near future.

Acknowledgements

The authors thank Masashi Sato (Kagawa University, Kagawa, Japan), Hisashi Ashida (Kindai University, Wakayama, Japan), and Donald K Ingram (Louisiana State University, Louisiana, USA) for valuable advice. This publication was partially supported by the Sasakawa Scientific Research Grant from The Japan Science Society [2018-6021].

Conflict of interest

The authors declare no competing financial interest. Tomoya Shintani is an employee of a private enterprise (Japan). However, the company provided no financial support for writing this book chapter.

Author details

Tomoya Shintani[1,2]*, Laura Lema-Perez[3] and Hideya Shintani[4]

1 Ehime University, Matsuyama, Japan

2 The Japanese Clinical Nutrition Association, Tokyo, Japan

3 Universidad Nacional de Colombia, Medellín, Colombia

4 Osaka Saiseikai Izuo Hospital, Osaka, Japan

*Address all correspondence to: shintanitomoya@gmail.com

References

[1] Martins I: Anti-Aging Genes Improve Appetite Regulation and Reverse Cell Senescence and Apoptosis in Global Populations. Advances in Aging Research 2016; 5: 9-26. DOI: 10.4236/aar.2016.51002.

[2] Martins I: Insulin Therapy and Autoimmune Disease with Relevance to Nonalcoholic Fatty Liver Disease. Non Alcoholic Fatty Liver Disease. An Update. IntechOpen. 2018.

[3] Harman D: Aging: A theory based on free radical and radiation chemistry. J Gerontol 1956; 11: 298-300.

[4] Peek CB, Levine DC, Cedernaes J, Taguchi A, Kobayashi Y, Tsai SJ, Bonar NA, McNulty MR, Ramsey KM, Bass J: Circadian Clock Interaction with HIF1α Mediates Oxygenic Metabolism and Anaerobic Glycolysis in Skeletal Muscle. Cell Metab 2017; 25: 86-92. DOI: 10.1016/j.cmet.2016.09.010.

[5] Zorov, Dmitry B et al: "Mitochondrial reactive oxygen species (ROS) and ROS-induced ROS release." Physiological reviews 2014; 94: 909-950. DOI:10.1152/physrev.00026.2013.

[6] Owusu-Ansah E, Banerjee: Reactive oxygen species prime Drosophila haematopoietic progenitors for differentiation. Nature 2009; 461: 537-541. DOI: https://doi.org/10.1038/nature08313

[7] Takeshige K, Minakami S: NADH- and NADPH dependent formation of superoxide anions by bovine heart submitochondrial particles and NADH ubiquinone reductase preparation. Biochem J 1979; 180: 129-135.

[8] Trumpower B L: The protonmotive Q cycle. Energy transduction by coupling of proton translocation to electron transfer by the cytochrome bc1 complex. J Biol Chem. 1990; 265: 11409-11412.

[9] McLennan HR, Degli Esposti M: The contribution for mitochondrial respiratory complexes to the production of reactive oxygen species. J Bioenerg Biomembr 2000; 32: 153-162.

[10] Forman HJ, Kennedy J: Dihydro orotate dependent superoxide production in rat brain and liver: a function of the primary dehydrogenase. Arch Biochem Biophys 1976; 173: 219-224.

[11] Tretter L, Adam-Vizi V: Generation of reactive oxygen species in the reaction catalyzed by α-ketoglutarate dehydrogenase. J Neurosci. 2004; 24: 7771-7778.

[12] Piotrowska A, Bartnik E: The role of reactive oxygen species and mitochondria in aging. Postepy Biochem. 2014; 60: 240-247.

[13] Ha H, Lee HB: Reactive oxygen species as glucose signaling molecules in mesangial cells cultured under high glucose. Kidney Int Suppl 2000; 77: S19-25. DOI: 10.1046/j.1523-1755.2000.07704.x.

[14] Mattson MP: Hormesis Defined. Ageing Research Reviews. 2007; 7: 1-7. DOI:10.1016/j.arr.2007.08.007.

[15] Rattan SI: Principles and practice of hormetic treatment of aging and age-related diseases. Human & Experimental Toxicology 2008; 27: 151-4. DOI:10.1177/0960327107083409

[16] Rattan, Suresh IS: Hormesis in aging. Ageing Research Reviews 2008; 7: 63-78. DOI:10.1016/j.arr.2007.03.002

[17] Gems D, Partridge L: "Stress-Response Hormesis and Aging: "That which Does Not Kill Us Makes Us Stronger"". Cell Metabolism 2008; 7: 200-203. DOI:10.1016/j.cmet.2008.01.001

[18] Kyriazis M: "Clinical Anti-Aging Hormetic Strategies". Rejuvenation Research 2005; 8: 96-100. DOI:10.1089/rej.2005.8.96

[19] Kyriazis M: "Practical applications of chaos theory to the modulation of human ageing: Nature prefers chaos to regularity". Biogerontology 2003; 4: 75-90. DOI:10.1023/A:1023306419861

[20] Ristow M, Zarse K: "How increased oxidative stress promotes longevity and metabolic health: The concept of mitochondrial hormesis (mitohormesis)". Experimental Gerontology 2010; 45: 410-8. DOI: 10.1016/j.exger.2010.03.014

[21] Lema-Perez L, Garcia-Tirado J, Builes-Montaño C, Alvarez H: Phenomenological-Based model of human stomach and its role in glucose metabolism. Journal of Theoretical Biology 2019; 460: 88-100.

[22] Mergenthaler P: "Sugar for the brain: the role of glucose in physiological and pathological brain function." Trends in neurosciences 2013; 36: 587-597. DOI:10.1016/j.tins.2013.07.001

[23] Ter H, Kasper W, Mireille JS: "Fructose Consumption, Lipogenesis, and Non-Alcoholic Fatty Liver Disease." Nutrients 2017; 9: 981. DOI:10.3390/nu9090981

[24] Abraham JD, Joseph K, David MW, editors. Handbook of Biodegradable Polymers. 1st ed. Boca Raton: CRC Press; 1998. 275p. ISBN: 978-1-4200-4936-7.

[25] Jens B, Christin H, Rebecca P, Yong D, Christa S-N: Association between random glucose and all-cause mortality: findings from the mortality follow-up of the German National Health Interview and Examination Survey 1998. BMC Endocr Disord 2018; 18: 95. DOI: 10.1186/s12902-018-0319-2.

[26] Carlos C: Chronic Hyperglycemia and Glucose Toxicity: Pathology and Clinical Sequelae. Postgraduate medicine 2012; 124: 90-7. DOI: 10.3810/pgm.2012.11.2615.

[27] Tappy L and Rosset R: Health outcomes of a high fructose intake: the importance of physical activity. J Physiol 2019; 597: 3561-3571. DOI: https://doi.org/10.1113/JP278246

[28] Barbieri M, Bonafe M, Franceschi C, Paolisso G: Insulin/IGF-I-signaling pathway: an evolutionarily conserved mechanism of longevity from yeast to humans. Am J Physiol Endocrinol Metab 2003; 285: E1064–E1071.

[29] Park YK, Yetley EA: Intakes and food sources of fructose in the United States. Am J Clin Nutr 1993; 58: 737S–747S.

[30] Gross S, Li L, Ford S, Liu S: Increased consumption of refined carbohydrates and the epidemic of type 2 diabetes in the United States: An ecologic assessment. Am. J Clin Nutr 2004; 79: 774-779.

[31] Martins I: "Sirtuin 1, a Diagnostic Protein Marker and its Relevance to Chronic Disease and Therapeutic Drug Interventions". EC Pharmacology and Toxicology 2018; 6; 209-215.

[32] Martins I: Single Gene Inactivation with Implications to Diabetes and Multiple Organ Dysfunction Syndrome. J Clin Epigenet 2017; 3: 24. DOI: 10.21767/2472-1158.100058

[33] Caton PW, Nayuni NK, Khan NQ, Wood EG, Corder R: Fructose induces gluconeogenesis and lipogenesis through a SIRT1-dependent mechanism. J Endocrinol 2011; 208: 273-283. DOI: 10.1530/JOE-10-0190.

[34] Collino M: High dietary fructose intake: Sweet or bitter life? World J Diabetes. 2011; 15: 77-81. DOI: 10.4239/wjd.v2.i6.77

[35] Ammam M, Fransaer J: Two-enzyme lactose biosensor based on β-galactosidase and glucose oxidase deposited by AC-electrophoresis: Characteristics and performance for lactose determination in milk. Sens. Actuators B Chem 2010; 148: 583-589.

[36] Acosta PB, Gross KC: "Hidden sources of galactose in the environment," European Journal of Pediatrics 1995; 154: S87–S92.

[37] Berry GT, Nissim I, Lin Z, Mazur AT, Gibson JB, and Segal S: "Endogenous synthesis of galactose in normal men and patients with hereditary galactosaemia," The Lancet 1995; 8982: 1073-1074.

[38] Lai K, Elsas JL, Wierenga JK: "Galactose toxicity in animals," IUBMB Life 2009; 61: 1063-1074.

[39] Yang ST, Silva EM: Novel products and new technologies for use of a familiar carbohydrate, milk lactose. J Dairy Sci 1995; 78: 2541-2562.

[40] Kretchmer N: Lactose and lactase. Sci Am 1972; 227: 70-79.

[41] Heyman MB: Lactose intolerance in infants, children, and adolescents. Pediatrics 2006, 118, 1279-1286.

[42] Dekker JP, Koenders D, Bruins JM: Lactose-free dairy products: Market developments, production, nutrition and health benefits. Nutriets 2019; 11: 551.

[43] Hodges KJ, Cao S, Cladis PD, Weaver MC: Lactose intolerance and bone health: The challenge of ensuring adequate calcium intake. Nutriets 2019; 11: 718.

[44] Nakanishi K, Matsuno R, Torii K, Yamamoto K, Kamikubo T: Properties of immobilized β-d-galactosidase from Bacillus circulans. Enzym Microb Technol 1983; 5: 115-120.

[45] Michaëlsson K, Wolk A, Langenskiöld S, Basu S, Lemming EW, Melhus H, Byberg L: Milk intake and risk of mortality and fractures in women and men: Cohort studies. BMJ 2014; 349: g6015.

[46] Lai K, Elsas LJ, Wierenga KJ: Galactose toxicity in animals. IUBMB Life 2009; 61: 1063-1074.

[47] Ho SC, Liu JH, Wu RY: Establishment of the mimetic aging effect in mice caused by D-galactose. Biogerontology 2003; 4: 15-18. DOI: https://doi.org/10.1023/A:1022417102206

[48] Azman KF, Zakaria R: d-Galactose-induced accelerated aging model: an overview. Biogerontology 2019; 20: 763-782. DOI: https://doi.org/10.1007/s10522-019-09837-y

[49] Lane M, Ingram DK, Roth G: 2-Deoxy-d-Glucose Feeding in Rats Mimics Physiologic Effects of Calorie Restriction. J Anti Aging Med 2009; 1: 327-337.

[50] Roth SG, Lane MA, Ingram DK: Caloric restriction mimetics: The next phase. Ann N Y Acad Sci 2005; 1057: 365-371.

[51] Wang A, Mouser J, Pitt J, Promislow D, Kaeberlein M: Rapamycin enhances survival in a Drosophila model of mitochondrial disease. Oncotarget 2016; 7: 80131-80139.

[52] Wan R, Camandola S, Mattson MP: Intermittent fasting and dietary supplementation with 2-deoxy-d-glucose improve functional and metabolic cardiovascular risk factors in rats. FASEB J 2003; 17: 1133-1134.

[53] Lee J, Bruce-Keller AJ, Kruman Y, Chan SL, Mattson MP: 2-Deoxy-d-glucose protects hippocampal neurons against excitotoxic and oxidative injury: Evidence for the involvement of stress proteins. J Neurosci Res 1999; 57: 48-61.

[54] Duan W, Mattson MP: Dietary restriction and 2-deoxyglucose administration improve behavioral outcome and reduce degeneration of dopaminergic neurons in models of Parkinson's disease. J Neurosci Res 1999; 57: 195-206.

[55] Singh S, Pandey S, Bhatt AN, Chaudhary R, Bhuria V, Kalra N, Soni R, Roy BG, Saluja D, Dwarakanath BS: Chronic dietary administration of the glycolytic inhibitor 2-deoxy-d-glucose (2-DG) inhibits the growth of implanted Ehrlich's ascites tumor in mice. PLoS ONE 2015; 10: e0132089.

[56] Priebe S, Menzel U, Zarse K, Groth M, Platzer M, Ristow M, Guthke R: Extension of life span by impaired glucose metabolism in *Caenorhabditis elegans* is accompanied by structural rearrangements of the transcriptomic network. Plos One 2013; 30: e77776.

[57] Minor RK, Smith DL, Sossong AM, Kaushik S, Poosala S, Spangler EL, Roth GS, Lane M, Allison DB. de Cabo R et al: Chronic ingestion of 2-deoxy-d-glucose induces cardiac vacuolization and increases mortality in rats. Toxicol. Appl. Pharmacol. 2010; 243: 332-339.

[58] Ingram DK, Roth GS, Lane MA, Ottinger MA, Zou S, de Cabo R, Mattison JA: The potential for dietary restriction to increase longevity in humans: extrapolation from monkey studies. Biogerontology 2006; 7: 143-148.

[59] Dark J, Miller DR, Zucker I: Reduced glucose availability induces torpor in Siberian hamsters. Am J Physiol 1994; 267: R496–R501.

[60] Wan R, Camandola S, Mattson MP: Intermittent fasting and dietary supplementation with 2-deoxy-D-glucose improve functional and metabolic cardiovascular risk factors in rats. FASEB J 2003; 17:1133-1134.

[61] Lane MA, Ingram DK, Roth GS: 2-Deoxy-D-glucose feeding in rats mimics physiological effects of calorie restriction. J Anti-Aging Med 1998;1: 327-337.

[62] Iida T, Hayashi N, Yamada T, Yoshikawa Y, Miyazato S, Kishimoto Y, Okuma K, Tokuda M, Izumori K: Failure of d-psicose absorbed in the small intestine to metabolize into energy and its low large intestinal fermentability in humans. Metabolism 2010; 59: 206-214.

[63] Mooradian AD, Smith M, Tokuda M: The role of artificial and natural sweeteners in reducing the consumption of table sugar: A narrative review. Clin Nutr ESPEN 2017; 18: 1-8.

[64] Hossain A, Yamaguchi F, Matsuo T, Tsukamoto I, Toyoda Y, Ogawa M, Nagata Y, Tokuda M: Rare sugar d-allulose: Potential role and therapeutic monitoring in maintaining obesity and type 2 diabetes mellitus. Pharmacol Ther 2015; 155: 49-59.

[65] Pongkan W, Jinawong, K., Pratchayasakul, W. et al: d-allulose provides cardioprotective effect by attenuating cardiac mitochondrial dysfunction in obesity-induced insulin-resistant rats. Eur J Nutr 2020; DOI: https://doi.org/10.1007/s00394-020-02394-y

[66] Pratchayasakul W, Jinawong K, Pongkan W, Jaiwongkam T, Arunsak B, Chunchai T, Tokuda M, Chattipakorn N, Chattipakorn CS: Not only metformin, but also D-allulose, alleviates metabolic disturbance and cognitive decline in prediabetic rats. Nutritional Neuroscience 2020: DOI: 10.1080/1028415X.2020.1840050

[67] Toyoda Y, Mori S, Umemura. N, Futamura N, Inoue H, Hata T, Miwa I, Murao K, Nishiyama A, Tokuda M: Suppression of blood glucose levels by d-psicose in glucose tolerance test in

diabetic rats. Jpn Pharmacol Ther 2010; 38: 261– 269.

[68] Ingram DK, Roth GS: Glycolytic inhibition: an effective strategy for developing calorie restriction mimetics. GeroScience 2020; DOI: https://doi.org/10.1007/s11357-020-00298-7

[69] Hayashi, N, Iida T, Yamada T, Okura K, Takehara I, Yamamoto T, Yamada K, Tokuda M: Study on the postprandial blood glucose suppression effect of d-psicose in borderline diabetes and the safety of long-term ingestion by normal human subjects. Biosci Biotechnol Biochem 2010; 74: 510-519.

[70] Kimura T, Kanasaki A, Hayashi N, Yamada T, Iida T, Nagata Y, Okuma K: d-Allulose enhances postprandial fat oxidation in healthy humans. Nutrition 2017; 43-44: 16-20.

[71] Han Y, Kwon EY, Yu M, Lee S, Kim HJ, Kim SB, Kim Y, Choi MS: A preliminary study for evaluating the dose-dependent effect of d-allulose for fat Mass reduction in adult humans: A randomized, double-blind, placebo-controlled trial. Nutrients 2018; 10:160. DOI: 10.3390/nu10020160.

[72] Reginster JY, Deroisy R, Rovati LC, Lee RL, Lejeune E, Bruyere O, Giacovelli G, Henrotin Y, Dacre JE, Gossett C: Long-term effects of glucosamine sulphate on osteoarthritis progression: A randomised, placebo-controlled clinical trial. Lancet 2001; 357: 251-256.

[73] Weimer S, Priebs J, Kuhlow D, Groth M, Priebe S, Mansfeld J, Merry TL, Dubuis S, Laube B, Pfeiffer AF et al: d-Glucosamine supplementation extends life span of nematodes and of ageing mice. Nat Commun 2014; 5: 3563.

[74] Tim JS, Kim Z, Anja V, Nadine U, Marc B, Michael R: Glucose restriction extends *Caenorhabditis elegans* life span by inducing mitochondrial respiration and increasing oxidative stress. Cell Metab 2007; 6: 280-293. DOI: 10.1016/j.cmet.2007.08.011.

[75] Barrientos C, Racotta R.; Quevedo L: Glucosamine attenuates increases of intraabdominal fat, serum leptin levels, and insulin resistance induced by a high-fat diet in rats. Nutr Res 2010; 30: 791-800.

[76] Katoh A, Kai H, Harada H, Niiyama H, Ikeda H: Oral administration of glucosamine improves vascular endothelial function by modulating intracellular redox state. Int. Heart J 2017; 58: 926-932.

[77] Pocobelli G, Kristal AR, Patterson RE, Potter JD, Lampe JW, Kolar A, Evans I, White E: Total mortality risk in relation to use of less-common dietary supplements. Am J Clin Nutr 2010; 91: 1791-1800.

[78] Zhi-Hao L, Xiang G, Vincent CHC et al: Associations of regular glucosamine use with all-cause and cause-specific mortality: a large prospective cohort study. Annals of the Rheumatic Diseases 2020; 79: 829-836.

[79] Metchnikoff E, Mitchell PC: The prolongation of life: optimistic studies. Putnam's Sons 1908, New York & London.

[80] Moskalev A, Chernyagina E, Kudryavtseva A, Shaposhnikov M: Geroprotectors: A Unified Concept and Screening Approaches. Aging Dis 2017; 8: 354-363. DOI: 10.14336/AD.2016.1022.

[81] Anisimov VN: Life span extension and cancer risk: myths and reality. Exp Gerontol 2001; 36: 1101-1136.

[82] Mills KF, Yoshida S, Stein LR, Grozio A, Kubota S, Sasaki Y, Redpath P, Migaud ME, Apte RS, Uchida K,

Yoshino J, Imai SI: Long-Term Administration of Nicotinamide Mononucleotide Mitigates Age-Associated Physiological Decline in Mice. Cell Metab 2016; 24:795-806. DOI: 10.1016/j.cmet.2016.09.013.

[83] Hubbard BP, Sinclair DA: Small molecule SIRT1 activators for the treatment of aging and age-related diseases. Trends Pharmacol Sci 2014; 35: 146-54. DOI: 10.1016/j.tips.2013.12.004.

[84] Anisimov VN, Popovich IG, Zabezhinski MA, Anisimov SV, Vesnushkin GM, Vinogradova IA: Melatonin as antioxidant, geroprotector and anticarcinogen. Biochim Biophys Acta 2006;1757:573-589. DOI: 10.1016/j.bbabio.2006.03.012.

[85] Boldyrev AA, Stvolinsky SL, Fedorova TN, Suslina ZA: Carnosine as a natural antioxidant and geroprotector: from molecular mechanisms to clinical trials. Rejuvenation Res 2010; 13: 156-158. DOI: 10.1089/rej.2009.0923.

Chapter 3

Impact of Sugar on Vision

Grace Ogbonna, Rosemary Ehigbo and Ogbonna Hannah

Abstract

Sugar forms an integral part of the human body, and contributes to normal body function. However, sugar in high quantities can be detrimental to the body especially to the eye. In the normal concentration, sugar in the form of glucose is found in the aqueous humour, and tears, and serves to provide nourishment to the avascular cornea, and lens respectively. Sugar at this stage may also be used to determine the post mortem interval of a cadaver. However, when in excess as may be seen in patients with diabetes, sugar can cause oxidative stress to the cornea, lens, and retina resulting in cornea oedema, cataract, retinal aneurysm which can contribute significantly to the prevalence of low vision, and vision impairment.

Keywords: sugar, cataract, oxidative stress, aneurysm

1. Introduction

Sugar forms an integral part of the human eye, and can be found in different parts of the eye including the tears, aqueous humour, and the lens. Its primary function in the eye includes; maintenance of the structural component of the eye, and the provision of nourishment to the surrounding structures of the eye wherein it is found. For instance, glucose found in the aqueous humour forms part of the required nourishment to the avascular lens, and cornea [1]. In the tears, sugar in the form of glucose forms part of the nutrients that supply the avascular cornea. The sugar in the vitreous is present as hyaluronic acid which is a molecular unit of glucusonite, and N-acetylglucosamine. Its function is to maintain the point of vitreous attachment to the retina. In general, sugar is important for the normal functioning of the human eye. In the lens, sugar is found as polysaccharides. Meyer *et al* [2] showed that there are at least three different polysaccharides in the cornea stroma - keratin sulfate, chondroitin-4-sulfate, and chondroitin, and may play a role in cornea healing.

Despite the role of sugar in maintaining the metabolic requirements of the human body, excessive sugar consumption can lead to high sugar concentration in blood circulation within the body system which can be detrimental to human health. Sustained high sugar level results in hyperglycaemia, and if left unchecked can result in Diabetes Mellitus. Diabetes mellitus is a group of metabolic diseases, characterized by chronic hyperglycaemia due to deficiency in the production, and/or usage of insulin. Diabetes mellitus can occur as either Type 1 (due to poor secretion of insulin) or Type 2 (due to poor usage of insulin for glucose metabolism).

Diabetes Mellitus presents with a myriad of ocular complications and has been identified as the leading cause of legal blindness globally. Complications secondary to diabetes affects almost every part of the eye and could result in diabetic retinopathy, cataracts, glaucoma, keratopathy, dry eye syndrome, and so many others (**Figure 1**).

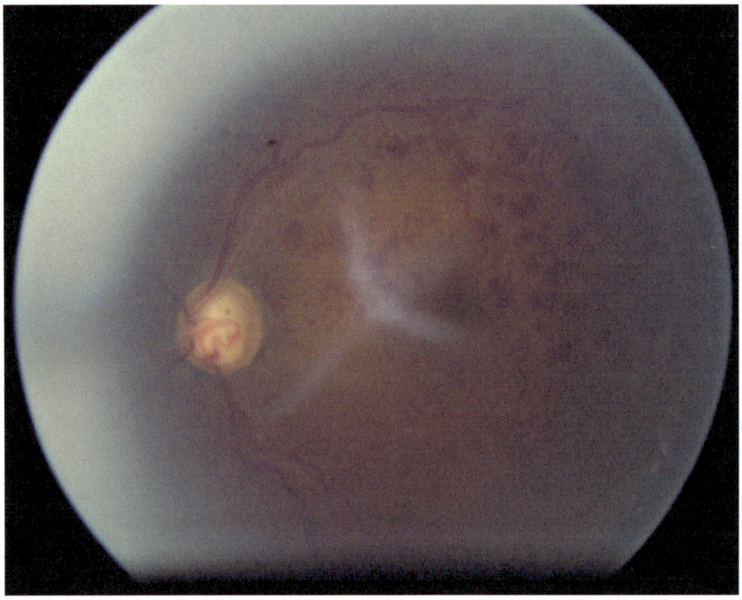

Figure 1.
Fundus picture of a proliferative diabetic retinopathy.

In recent years, diabetes mellitus has become a serious public health concern as the number of diabetic patients worldwide has more than doubled over the last three decades. In 2010, 286 million people were said to be diabetic, and this was projected to increase to 439 million by 2030 [3]. As the prevalence of DM, duration, and onset increases, the number of patients with ocular complications due to the condition is also expected to increase.

2. Mechanism of action of the effect of hyperglycaemic on the eyes

The mechanism of action of hyperglycaemia on the eyes and the consequential damage to the eyes have been likened to that of the effect of ageing on the eye [4]. Various factors such as pro-inflammation, oxidative stress, glycosylated cross-linkages, the formation of advanced glycelated end-products (AGE), vascular permeability, vascular endothelial growth factor (VEGF), and epigenetic factors have been found to cause to ageing changes in the eye. Similarly, these factors have been implicated in the development of ocular complications secondary to sustained increased sugar levels in the body [5–7].

Further, Insulin resistance as may be seen in diabetic patients has been associated with the repression of a Sirtuin 1(Sirt 1) [8], which is the gene responsible for the regulation of appetite in the geriatric population. Sirt 1 is also known as the anti-ageing gene due to its ability to alleviate oxidative stress [8–10]. Repression of Sirt 1 gene may lead to mitochondrial apoptosis, and in diabetic patients can also lead to diabetic retinopathy due to oxidative stress [8, 10, 11].

3. Sugar, and the lens: an overview

The human crystalline lens is the structure directly behind the iris, and in front of the vitreous humour [1]. The lens thickness and curvature allows it to contribute significantly to refraction [12]. It is also responsible for accommodation in non-presbyopic, and pre-presbyopic people. Its transparent nature allows for the passage of light to the retina. Physiologically, the lens contains 2/3 water, and 1/3 protein (water-soluble and water-insoluble proteins) [13]. Water-soluble proteins are responsible for maintaining the lens optical properties. On the other hand, water-insoluble protein maintains cellular structures, architectural arrangement, and alignment.

The lens lacks blood vessel supplies to it and is therefore regarded as avascular. Due to the lack of blood vessels in the lens, it acquires most of its nutrition from the aqueous humour, through the aerobic glycolysis, or through the pentose phosphate pathway (sorbitol pathway). The sorbitol pathway is believed to be a pathway through which glucose, and galactose from the aqueous humour is absorbed into the lens [14]. When glucose is absorbed, it is reduced to sorbitol by the aldose reductase enzyme. Further to this, sorbitol is metabolized by the sorbitol dehydrogenase, whereas galacititol remains in the lens nearly not metabolized for a prolonged period. In diabetes, the increased presence of sugar in the blood results in increased glucose level in the aqueous, therefore bringing about increased sugar inflow into the lens through the sorbitol pathway [15]. Unfortunately, the sorbitol is produced faster than it is converted to fructose by the sorbitol dehydrogenase. This, therefore, means an increased amount of sorbitol in the lens. The prolonged presence of sorbitol in the lens results in increased intracellular fluid as a response to increased osmotic pressure, therefore causing the swelling of the lens material. Further, because sorbitol is polar, it is hardly removed from the lens through simple diffusion.

3.1 Sugar, and cataract

Sustained hyperglycaemia causes the inflow of sugar into the lens resulting in the swelling of the lens material. This also results in the loss of the lens structural arrangement (lens fibres), precipitation of the water-insoluble proteins, oxidation of the water-insoluble proteins, hardening of the lens fibres, formation of permanent bonds, and eventually cataract.

Sugar induced cataract is a common occurrence, and a significant cause of visual impairment among diabetic patients. According to the Framingham study findings, diabetic patients under 65 are four times more likely to develop cataracts than their normal age mates. The onset of cataract in diabetes is often associated with fluctuations in the sugar level of a sufferer, and the cataract progresses rapidly once initiated. Even though the process of cataract formation in a diabetic patient is known, however, there is no known mechanism to delay its formation in the presence of Hyperglycaemic [16]. Nevertheless, cataract surgery is a recommended, and effective way of manageing diabetic cataracts.

Early cataract extraction in diabetic patients though recommended, should be approached with caution, and is advisable to be done with regulated blood sugar levels as healing may be delayed due to Hyperglycaemic [17, 18]. Although, a study in Nigeria reported no significant difference in the visual outcome of diabetic patients post-cataract when compared to age-matched nondiabetic controls, however, complications such as rubeosis, acceleration in the formation of retinopathy, post-operative inflammation,, and incidence of clinical, and angiographic cystoid oedema has been reported to occur more in diabetic patients following cataract extraction [19]. Given these complications, the preferred method of cataract extraction in diabetic patients is phacoemulsification as this has been associated with fewer complications, and better prognosis.

3.2 Sugar, and refractive error

Refractive changes have been noted to occur in diabetic patients. A number of earlier clinical studies had reported an association between sustained hyperglycaemia, and refractive shift towards increased myopia [12, 19, 20]. Myopic shift occurs when a diabetic patient experiences more myopia than the regular refractive error status. This happens due to an increase in the inflow of sugar into the lens through the sorbitol pathway catalysed by the aldose reductase activity [21, 22]. People with diabetes have been observed to have a higher prevalence of myopia compared to those without diabetes [23]. In a study conducted by Jacobsen *et al* [24] it was determined that the prevalence of myopia (spherical equivalent 0.5 D) was 53.3% among 252 type 1 diabetic patient age 16–26 years old. The relative risk of a myopic shift was determined to be 1.7 in patients aged 16–21 years, and 1.6 in patients with HbA1c above 8.8%. Insulin dosage was not related to myopia. Klein et al. [21] showed that persons of similar age with T1D were likely to be more myopic than those with T2D. In general, myopia associated with diabetes reverses when sugar control is instituted.

Although past studies had reported a myopic shift in refractive status following an increase in sugar level, however, recent studies have also noted a hyperopic shift associated with glycaemic control [25, 26]. Hyperopic shift following hyperglycaemia control has been reported to occur when glucose levels fall a few days or weeks after the initiation of glycaemic control [12, 27]. This hyperopia was associated with increased lens thickness, and a decrease in anterior chamber depth [22]. Lin *et al* [12] reported the development of hyperopia in 4 men and 1 woman who was treated with insulin. According to their report, the hyperopia peaked at 11.7 days after initiation of glycaemic control and tapered off at 64.0 days after treatment initiation. From this it can be deduced that institution of treatment in diabetic patients is often followed by two refractive changes; one involving a rapid refractive change towards the direction of hyperopic, and the other is a gradual change to the patient's normal refractive status.

In general, both myopic, and hyperopic shifts are transient, and patients' refractive status gradually returns to the baseline values a few days or weeks after sugar stabilizes. Thus, it can be said that both myopic, and hyperopic shift may occur with changes in sugar levels in a hyperglycemic patient [25]. Hence, change in prescription glasses should be approached with caution as glasses prescribed during this time will only be durable during the said sugar fluctuations [28].

3.3 Sugar, and accommodation

Several studies have reported on biometric changes such as lens thickening, increase in the lens surface curvature and a decrease in the refractive index secondary to diabetes [29]. According to Mathebula, and Makunyane "people with diabetes have accelerated age-related biometric ocular changes compared to people without diabetes" [4]. Elevated sugar levels in pre-presbyopic patients have been associated with a reduction in the amplitude of accommodation. According to Huntjens and O'Donnell, amplitude of accommodation is lower in people living with Type I patients than that of their non-diabetic age-matched, even in the absence of non-detectable retinal damage [25].

Amplitude of accommodation is important for maintaining images on the retina while doing near work. A reduction in amplitude of accommodation means that the near point becomes receded, and a patient will have difficulties reading things at near as seen in presbyopic patients. This has unfortunately been found in pre-presbyopic diabetic patients who show signs of presbyopia earlier than their age match nondiabetic counterparts. The effect of hyperglycaemia on the accommodative system may be due to changes in lens glucose metabolism, ischemic hypoxia on the oculomotor nerve, and ciliary muscles. Some studies have noted that the longer the duration of diabetes, the more likely the reduction in the amplitude of accommodation.

4. Sugar, and the cornea

The cornea is a superficial organ most affected by high sugar levels [30]. The impact of sugar on the cornea varies with its level and duration, and may underpin specific systemic complications that may be associated with diabetes. At normal glycaemic levels, sugar serves as one of the dissolved nutrients in the tears, and aqueous humour that nourishes the cornea. Sugar is also found in the cornea stroma in the form of polysaccharides (glycosaminoglycan GAG) [31]. GAG reduces the effects of diffraction when light is directed towards the eye. Chondroitin sulphate an element that plays a role in cornea wound healing is also made from polysaccharides.

However, in diabetes, sugar promises to be detrimental to the anatomical and physiological wellbeing of the cornea. Structural components such as the epithelium, the nerves, immune cells, and the endothelium of the cornea are often negatively affected. Sustained hyperglycaemia reduces cornea sensitivity and innervation due to peripheral neuropathy. These nerve alterations occur all over the cornea including at the cornea scleral junction (limbal region) where new epithelial cells are formed [31]. When there is a reduction in corneal sensitivity, affected patients experiences various symptoms, and in most cases become susceptible to further damages to the eye. Reduction in corneal sensitivity has been identified as a predictor for the development of peripheral neuropathy in diabetic patients.

Other cornea complications such as corneal infections, ulcers, and oedema have been reported in diabetic patients with poorly controlled glycaemic levels. Sugar induced cornea swelling increases the fragility of the cornea epithelium and can result in stroma oedema [32]. This for unknown reasons affects the stromal collagen bundles and increases corneal autofluorescence level. The variation between the normal fluorescence level and increased autofluorescence in the corneal may be an indicator of changed corneal metabolism due to impaired corneal mitochondria metabolism. Corneal fluorescence may also be an indicator of a pathological breakdown of the blood-aqueous- barrier as may be seen in patients with proliferative diabetic retinopathy.

Sustained hyperglycaemic levels in the body also increases the chances of corneal erosions, persistent epithelial defects, corneal endothelial damage, and dry eye [6, 22, 32]. With Sustained hyperglycaemia the cornea faces difficulties with wound healing, and most times there is incomplete wound healing, thus small corneal erosions become persistent as wound healing is delayed. Delayed wound healing has been linked to a reduction in cornea epithelium regeneration secondary to a decrease in cornea sensitivity, which occurs as a result of peripheral neuropathy [6]. linked Further, because the ability of the cornea to ward off infections is reduced, infections like fungal keratitis occurs and remains recurrent [33].

5. Sugar, and the lids, and conjunctiva

The lids and conjunctiva are tissues in the body that protects the eye against external invaders. Sustained high blood sugar level increases the susceptibility of the human system to bacterial infection. In the lid, this susceptibility leads to a recurrent bacterial infection which can lead to the formation of stye, and blepharitis.

High sugar and reduced insulin as is obtainable in diabetes pose damaging consequences to the meibomian gland. Like other sebaceous glands, insulin forms an essential component for the optimal functioning of the sebaceous glands and resistance or reduction in its absorption results in the dysfunction of the Meibomian gland. Similarly, sustained increase in sugar level brings about the lipolysis of adipocytes, this, therefore, means that sustained sugar levels in the Meibomian gland will reduce the quality of the meibum secreted in the eye. Meibum is the secretion responsible for ensuring the liquid part of the tears (aqueous) does not overflow or evaporate, hence reduction in the quality of meibum would allow for tear evaporation, bringing about dry eye effect in diabetic patients.

Similarly, the goblet cells found in the conjunctiva which are responsible for the production of the mucin layer of the tear film are often adversely affected with Hyperglycaemic. Diabetes also affects the conjunctival blood vessels in similar ways as it does to the retinal blood vessels [34]. In the conjunctiva, capillary loss, and microvascular dilatation had similarly been observed as a consequence of sustained hyperglycemia. Similarly, studies have reported on the tortuosity of conjunctival blood vessels.

6. Sugar, and dry eye

Dry eye is a disorder of the tear film which results in symptoms such as pain, burning, itchiness, stinging, grittiness, foreign body sensation, tearing, and ocular fatigue. Due to the multifactorial nature of dry eye onset, it has been referred to as a disease of the lacrimal function unit (LFU). The lacrimal function unit is made up of the cornea, lid, conjunctiva, Meibomian gland, the sensory, and the motor nerves which all work as a unit to maintain the tear film layer. Dry eye is a common experience in diabetic patients.

The occurrence of dry eye in a diabetic patient may be as a result of the negative effect of hyperglycaemia on any part of the lacrimal function unit. For instance, insufficient production of tears due to reduced cornea sensitivity secondary to autonomic neuropathy has been blamed as part of the reason for dry eye development in diabetic patients [35]. Corneal sensitivity forms part of the neuronal loophole feedback mechanism for reflex tear secretion. Autonomic neuropathy affects the nerves that control the lacrimal gland secretion, bringing about a reduction in tears secretion, due to reduced corneal sensitivity. For instance, damage to the microvasculature of the lacrimal gland accompanied by autonomic neuropathy in diabetic patients often impairs lacrimation, therefore, resulting in dry eye symptoms in such a patient. The reduction in tear secretion accounts for the low Schirmer test result as may be seen in diabetic patients. It is noteworthy that once corneal peripheral neuropathy sets in, corneal sensitivity starts and the magnitude of reflex tear secretion is affected.

Also, dry eye may result due to a reduction in the population density of the goblet cells secondary to the effect of diabetes on the cells on the goblet cell function [22]. The goblet cells are responsible for the secretion of mucin which is the first layer of the tear film. The mucin layer is responsible for maintaining the tear film layer on the cornea to avoid the drying out of the cornea and maintaining its lustre. Therefore, a reduction in the density of the goblet cells will bring about a decrease in the secretion of the mucin layer, resulting in the inability of the tear film to remain stable on the cornea. Also, alongside the reduction in goblet cell density, there is an accompanying reduction in the ability of the mucin layer to "pickup-up' the cytology impression necessary to maintain the tear film spreading, and stability on the cornea. These two factors (goblet cell density, and mucin sensitivity), have been cited to partly be responsible for the reduction in the tear break-up time.

Some retinal changes, and procedures have similarly been linked with dry eye in patients with prolonged, and sustained hyperglycaemia. Reduction in total tear secretion has been reported in patients with non-proliferative diabetic retinopathy. This on the other hand is relatively small in people without retinopathy. Also, pan-retinal photocoagulation has been suggested to increase dry eye syndrome in patients.

Dry eye symptoms in diabetic patients are often associated with longer duration of the disease; it may also be associated with glycaemic level (HBA1c) [36]. Further, poorly controlled glycaemic level has been associated with more symptoms of dry eye. The most frequently encountered dry eye disease symptoms in diabetic patients include itching, burning, and foreign body sensation. Detection of dry eye in a diabetic patient can be achieved through conducting a comprehensive eye examination, which among others should measure the volume of tears, and determine the quality of the tears. This can be achieved by running specific diagnostic tests such as the Tear Film Break-Up Time (TFBUT), fluoresce test, Schirmer test, and rose Bengal. Management of dry eye in patients with diabetes strongly revolves around glycaemic control, and healthy lifestyle.

7. Sugar, and the iris

Hyperglycaemia affects the iris in various ways. Morphologically, changes in the iris structure, vessels, pigment granules, and vacuolation of the pigment. The iris epithelium due to hyperglycaemia can experience depigmentation of the cells which often deposits on the corneal endothelium or is washed by the aqueous flow to the trabecular meshwork where it could block the outflow of aqueous from the meshwork, therefore resulting in the building of ocular tension (increased intraocular pressure). Also, Hyperglycaemic may cause rubeosis iridis (the formation abnormal blood vessels on the epithelial layer of the iris), a response that has been associated with ischaemia secondary to retinal capillary dropout.

Further, abnormal iris transilluminance has been reported to occur in type 2 diabetes patients. This has been associated with short term retinopathy and is said to be an indicator or marker for rapidly progressive retinopathy in diabetes [37]. Similarly, ultrastructural changes have been reported in the regions of the sphincter, and dilator muscles of the iris, with more of the changes seen in the iris, this may explain why the pupil in diabetic patient's experience miosis while in dark rooms.

8. Sugar, and the vitreous

In the presence of hyperglycaemia, the vitreous gel and vitreous interface experiences alterations which are often predictors to the development of diabetic retinopathy. Changes in the vitreous gel due to diabetic mellitus may include; increased collagen fibril cross-linking, accumulation of advanced glycation end products, liquidation of the vitreous gels, vitreous haemorrhage and alteration in the concentration of various proteins present in the vitreous [38, 39]. In some cases, there may also be the development of new vessel on the vitreous surface, this can happen in response to retinal ischemia and can result in a structural change in the vitreous [40, 41]. The presence of severe non-clearing vitreous haemorrhage may be an indicator for the.

9. Sugar, and the retina

Sugar affects different layers of the retina, and in most cases is very detrimental, and can lead to blindness. Diabetic retinopathy is the most common cause of visual impairment in patients living with diabetes.

9.1 Sugar, and diabetic retinopathy

Diabetic retinopathy is a microvascular complication of diabetes. It is said to occur to some degree in almost all type 1 diabetic patients and in nearly 77% of people living with type 2 diabetes for more than 2 decades [7]. Its formation has been linked to hyperglycaemic induced electrolyte imbalance secondary to high aldose reductase levels in the retina [39]. The electrolyte imbalance leads to the loss of retinal endothelial cells and loss of vascular pericytes which are responsible for regulating the retinal vascular tone. Loss of endothelial cells results in the breakdown of the blood-retinal-barrier resulting in an increase in the vascular permeability. On the other hand, the loss of the pericytes results in vasodilation and the thickening of the capillary basement membrane all of which leads to microaneurysm (formation of small outpouchings from blood vessel walls) [42], a primary indicator of early retinopathy changes in diabetes [43].

There are different stages of diabetic retinopathy: mild non-proliferative diabetic retinopathy, pre-proliferative diabetic retinopathy, and proliferative diabetic retinopathy. According to the findings of the Wisconsin study, the prevalence of retinopathy in patients with diabetes increases from 2% to 97.5% in people with diabetes less than 2 years, and 15 or more years respectively. Prevalence of proliferative retinopathy was notably at zero but increased with age to 4%, 25%, and 67% among diabetic patients who had lived with diabetes for 10 years, 15 years, and 35 years respectively. Proliferative diabetic retinopathy is the most complicated stage of diabetic retinopathy and is often associated with other complications such as vitreous haemorrhage, tractional retinal detachment, combined tractional rhegmatogenous retinal detachment, and severe fibrovascular proliferation.

Proliferative diabetic retinopathy is said to occur due to prolonged retinal ischemia secondary to Hyperglycaemic. Retinal ischemia leads to the production of angiogenic factors which are produced in an attempt for the retina to revascularize the hypoxic areas of the retina. Thus the release of angiogenic factors is the retinal way of seeking for a secondary means of transporting oxygen to the affected parts of the retina. After the formation of the angiogenic factor, there appears to be an interaction between the angiogenic factors, and the vascular endothelial growth factor (VEGF) thereby inducing the growth of new blood vessels (neovascularization). The new vessels are fragile, and can easily rupture, but they proliferate persistently. The proliferation of the new blood vessels is accompanied by varying degrees of fibrous tissue proliferation. Fibrous tissue proliferation into the vitreoretinal interface brings about the formation of fibrovascular membranes in the vitreoretinal interface.

The fibrovascular tissues attach themselves to the vitreoretinal interface focally (at a point) or broadly (at different points). The point of attachment of the fibrovascular tissue to the vitreoretina exerts tractional forces at these points, therefore, pulling on the retina, and resulting in tractional retinal detachment.

Although the duration and glycaemic control play a role in the development of retinopathy, genetics, and individual disparity contribute significantly to the development and degree of retinopathy. Diabetic retinopathy has been cited to occur more globally in Latin Americans, and South Asians [5]. Clustering of diabetic retinopathy among people of similar ethnicity suggests that genetics could play a significant role in its development. The role of familial genetics in the development of diabetic retinopathy was demonstrated by Leslie and Pyke who found that 95% of concordant type 2 diabetic twins versus 68% of concordant type 1 diabetic identical twins develop a similar degree of diabetic retinopathy. Also, siblings with diabetes have similar levels of diabetes when compared to other levels of retinopathies seen in non-family members. Familial clustering for the risk of developing severe retinopathy to increase among those who have diabetic relatives with positive retinopathy with an odds ratio of 5.4 compared to those whose relatives do not have the retinopathy [44].

Further, the genes responsible for encoding the aldose reductase (ALR), Angiotensin-1-converting enzyme, endothelial nitric oxide synthase (eNOS), a receptor for advanced glycation end products (RAGE), and Vascular Endothelial Growth Factor (VEGF), has been implicated in the development of Diabetic retinopathy [44]. Also, evidence exist which suggest that low-grade inflammatory responses underlies the resultant vascular complications seen in diabetes retinopathy. This, therefore, implies that diabetic retinopathy is an inflammatory disease that results due to elevated systemic cytokines like TNF-a, and IL-1B, and elevated numbers of activated leukocytes circulating in the retinal blood vessels.

The role of angiotensin II in the formation of diabetic retinopathy has been well studied with most studies promoting possible retardation of the proliferation process seen in diabetic retinopathy through the use of drugs that blocks the renin-angiotensin system. This is because angiotensin II which promotes vascular remodelling, and proliferation can cause an increase in the growth of capillaries, and cell permeability, and oxidative stress which is common in the formation of diabetic retinopathy.

The role of vasodilators like nitric oxide has rather been inconclusive, and a matter of debate. While some researchers believe that nitric oxide could lead to retinal damage and death, some others believe that nitric oxide enzyme may be protective in the development of diabetic retinopathy. Also, the actions of Glucagon-Like-Peptide-1 (GLP-1) a 30-amino acid, which is a hormone produced in the intestine, and helps in regulating blood glucose has been found to play a protective role on the retinal cells via the reduction of oxidative stress on the retina, which is protective in the development of diabetic retinopathy [11]. The action of GLP-1 is often activated by SIRT1 an anti-ageing gene.

10. Sugar and the optic disc, and nerve

Sustained sugar level affects the optic nerve resulting in nerve abnormalities, for instance, the optic disc often experiences pronounced oxidative stress, ischaemia, and neurodegeneration which eventually results into loss of the retinal nerve fibre layer, and optic atrophy. Optic atrophy may occur due to the inability of the nerves to access nourishment secondary to hyperglycaemia. Optic atrophy secondary to hyperglycaemia is very common in diabetic patients who are in their fourth decade of life. Although this presents no symptoms, it requires constant monitoring as it may ensure to proliferative diabetic retinopathy.

Optic nerve atrophy may also occur as a result of damage following photocoagulation treatment. This often shows a characteristics appearance that is abnormal which may or may not be similar to glaucomatous damage [45]. This is due to nerve damage that may be associated with the destruction of the axons of the retinal ganglion cells following pan-retinal photocoagulation. Other causes of optic atrophy may include previous diabetic papilopathy, nonarteritic ischemic neuropathy, and multiple nerve fibre layer infarcts.

Neovascularization at the optic disc head may also occur especially in the proliferative stage of diabetes. Although the formation of these vessels are mechanisms by which the eye seems to transport oxygen to areas without nourishment, however, the new vessels formed are both fragile, and vulnerable to rupture, hence presents a danger to the eye.

11. Diabetes induced maculopathy

Diabetes induced maculopathy is a common occurrence in people with diabetic retinopathy [41]. Its prevalence is often determined by the type of diabetes, the severity of diabetic retinopathy, and duration of the disease. Type 1 diabetic patients are less likely to develop maculopathy, than type 2 diabetic patients [40]. Also, the occurrence of maculopathy in type 1 diabetic patients is highly dependent on the duration of the disease. Most of the patients with type 1 diabetes will rarely develop maculopathy before 8 years of the disease, with about 25–30% developing maculopathy after 20 years of the disease [41, 43]. About 3% of type 2 diabetic patients with non-proliferative retinopathy will have macular oedema, whereas between 40%, and 70% of those with moderate, and proliferative retinopathy respectively would end up developing macular oedema. Among this population, nearly half of them will experience fovea involvement of the macula oedema [43].

12. Pupil involvement in diabetes

Pupillary involvement is a common occurrence in diabetic patients and has been suggested to be due to autonomic neuropathy secondary to degenerative changes at the nerve terminal. In the pupil, the autonomous nervous system regulates the sphincter, and dilator muscles which controls the pupillary response to light, accommodation, and drugs. Sustained high sugar level often results in autonomic neuropathy which meant that nerves lose their ability to respond or conduct sensations as they ought to. The occurrence of autonomic neuropathy results in partial denervation of mostly the dilator muscle of the pupil. This, therefore, implies different pupillary responses to normal pupillary stimulus diabetic patients will be affected. For instance, diabetic pupils have excessive miotic pupils in dim illumination, also diabetic pupils experience loss of light reflex, non-syphilitic-Argy Robertson pupil has been reported. Further, variations in response to topical mydriatic agents have similarly been noted.

13. Sugar, and glaucoma

There are still conflicting opinions regarding the relationship between glaucoma and diabetes, however, the mechanism that leads to the autonomic dysfunction in the regulation of intraocular pressure, fluctuation of intraocular pressure, and the increased susceptibility of retinal ganglion cells to cell death can easily be rationalized [46]. According to Negi and Vernon [43], diabetic patients are at high risk of developing higher intraocular pressures than their non-diabetic counterparts. Proliferative diabetes is one of the leading causes of neovascular glaucoma.

14. Sugar, and ophthalmoplegia

Ophthalmoplegia is a rare adverse effect of diabetes mellitus. It is often associated with multiple cranial nerve palsies affecting nerve III, IV, and VI. Patients with ophthalmoplegia secondary to diabetes often make a full recovery after 12 weeks of the onset of the condition [47]. A study by Kahtani et al. [48] reported ophthalmoplegia to be more common in male than female diabetic patients. Medial squint and Ptosis have also been reported in patients with acute vasculitis due to diabetes mellitus.

15. Sugar, and low vision

Complications secondary to diabetes mellitus is the leading cause of blindness in developed countries [6, 40]. According to global estimates, 5% of the 37 million cases of blindness occur secondary to diabetic retinopathy [7]. However, not all cases of diabetic retinopathy results in blindness, some others cause low vision in affected patients.

Low vision as defined by World Health Organization (WHO), is the visual acuity of less than 6/18 in the best-corrected eye of a patient. It can also be defined as the visual field of less than 10 degrees in a patient. There exists a strong relationship between complications resulting from sustained hyperglycaemia as seen in diabetes and low vision. Some of the complications resulting from hyperglycaemia brings about visual changes in sufferers which may eventually lead to low vision. Some visual changes that have been reported by hyperglycaemic patients include changes in Visual acuity, colour vision, contrast sensitivity, reduction in glare tolerance, and visual field all, of which affects a person's quality of life.

15.1 Sugar, and visual acuity

Because visual acuity status is affected by the status of the retina, cornea, lens, and the anterior chamber, visual acuity is one of the visual functions that is heavily affected by hyperglycaemia at different stages of the disease. Visual acuity may be affected by the presence of Diabetic cataract, which reduces the clarity of the lens. Visual acuity may also be affected by the presence of retinopathy which results in irreversible damage in the visual threshold of the patient. Other causes of reduction in visual acuity in a diabetic patients patient may include macular oedema, corneal haze, variations in the refractive status of the eyes due to variations in glycaemic levels, and procedures such as photocoagulation for diabetic macular oedema [49].

15.2 Sugar, and colour vision

Acquired dyschromatopsia has been reported to be common in people living with type 2 diabetes. The Okubo colour study, conducted among type diabetic patients showed that there is an-increased-adjusted-odds (5.89) for the development of colour vision impairment by type 2 diabetic compared with their age-matched normal glycaemic peers [2]. Some studies have reported an increase in the incidence of acquired, non-sex-linked blue-yellow colour vision deficit in diabetic patients. According to a study by Melisa et al., the blue-yellow colour deficit is more pronounced as diabetic retinopathy progresses, and is worse among patients who may have undergone laser treatment. The association between colour vision deficit and diabetes may be because diabetes irrespective of stage gradually affects the optic nerve as well as the retina, therefore resulting in abnormalities. Tan et al. also showed that more than 6 duration of type two diabetes may predispose patients to develop colour vision impairment [50].

15.3 Sugar and contrast sensitivity

Contrast sensitivity is a measure of the amount of contrast required to detect or recognize a visual target. It is a very important visual function in a person. Unfortunately, contrast sensitivity has been reported to decline with sustained hyperglycaemia. This has been attributed to retinal neurosensorial losses which may precede the occurrence of retinopathy in diabetic patients [51]. According to studies by Alberto et al. the occurrence of reduced contrast sensitivity is more in type 1 diabetic patients with retinopathy than with those without retinopathy [52]. Reduced contrast sensitivity can also be found in patients with type 2 diabetes. Safi *et al.* showed that contrast sensitivity decline was aggravated with the progression of retinopathy [53].

15.4 Sugar and visual field

Visual field defects have been reported as one of the notable low vision abnormalities that can occur in diabetic patients. Patrick and Lavin reported the occurrence of reversible homonymous hemianopia caused by non-ketotic hyperglycaemia in four patients with type 2 diabetes mellitus. [54]. Their report also noted that among the patients, homonymous hemianopia was the first manifestation of diabetes mellitus type 2 in two of the patients. Other factors such cerebrovascular accident, coexisting glaucoma, and pan-retinal photocoagulation has been reported as reasons for visual field defects in diabetic patients [43].

Visual processing disorders may also be seen in diabetic patients following cerebrovascular accident. Processing defects such as visual neglect and extinction has been reported to be partially reversible in these patients following treatment, and interventions.

16. Role of vitreous sugar in the determination of post-mortal interval

Sugar in the vitreous has found its usefulness in forensic medicine, where it can be used to determine the time of death and possible causes of death. The fact that there are biochemical changes in the blood glucose pathway after death makes the use of blood glucose in the biochemical analysis of the state of a cadaver difficult [55]. However, this difficulty can be overcome if the vitreous humor is used, given that, it is better preserved after death. Use of the concentration of sugar in the vitreous to determine the time of death has gradually gained some level of acceptance in forensic medicine and has been determined to have major advantages over other body fluids. Some of its advantages include its accessibility and the fact that after death it is often protected against putrefaction.

17. Effect of low sugar intake on vision

Although most of the emphasis of the impact of sugar in the eye is often placed on high sugar level, however low sugar level can also be detrimental to the eye.

The impact of low sugar level includes blurred vision, reduced contrast sensitivity, and central scotomas [56, 57].

18. Conclusions

Sugar forms a component part of the eye. Its presence at normal concentration is very important for the normal visual function, however when low or high, sugar can have very negative impact on vision.

Conflict of interest

The authors declare no conflict of interest.

Author details

Grace Ogbonna[1*], Rosemary Ehigbo[2] and Ogbonna Hannah[3]

1 Mzuzu University, Mzuzu, Malawi

2 Specialist Hospital Umuahia, Umuahia, Abia State, Nigeria

3 Umudike College of Agriculture, Umuahia, Nigeria

*Address all correspondence to: ogbonnagrace19@gmail.com

References

[1] Chakrabarti A. Posterior capsular rent: Genesis and management. Posterior Capsul Rent Genes Manag. 2017;1-279.

[2] Shoji T, Sakurai Y, Sato H, Chihara E, Takeuchi M. Do type 2 diabetes patients without diabetic retinopathy or subjects with impaired fasting glucose have impaired colour vision? The Okubo Color Study Report. Diabet Med. 2011;28(7):865-871.

[3] Burda N. The Incidence of Dry Eye Disease Related to Long Term Diabetes Mellitus Tip 2. Juniper Online J Case Stud. 2017;1(5):5-8.

[4] Mathebula SD, Makunyane PS. Amplitude of accommodation is reduced in pre-presbyopic diabetic patients. J Endocrinol Metab Diabetes South Africa. 2017;22(1):64-68.

[5] Jeng-Miller KW, Baumal CR. Genetics of Diabetic Retinopathy. Current Management of Diabetic Retinopathy. Elsevier Inc.; 2018. 37-40 p.

[6] Han SB, Yang HK, Hyon JY. Influence of diabetes mellitus on anterior segment of the eye. Clin Interv Aging. 2019;14:53-63.

[7] Lee C, Adler AI. Epidemiologic Evidence on Antioxidant-related Micronutrients and Diabetic Retinopathy. Diabetes: Oxidative Stress and Dietary Antioxidants. Elsevier; 2013. 231-236 p.

[8] Martins IJ. populations Current Updates in Gerontology Geriatric Medicine and Heat Shock Gene Therapy in Global Populations. 2016;1-5.

[9] Martins IJ. Anti-Aging Genes Improve Appetite Regulation and Reverse Cell Senescence and Apoptosis in Global Populations. 2016;(January):9-26.

[10] Zhou M, Luo J, Zhang H. Role of Sirtuin 1 in the pathogenesis of ocular disease (Review). 2018;13-20.

[11] Karbasforooshan H, Karimi G. Biomedicine & Pharmacotherapy The role of SIRT1 in diabetic retinopathy. Biomed Pharmacother. 2018;97(October 2017):190-194.

[12] Lin SF, Lin PK, Chang FL, Tsai RK. Transient hyperopia after intensive treatment of hyperglycemia in newly diagnosed diabetes. Ophthalmologica. 2009;223(1):68-71.

[13] Lund AL, Smith JB, Smith DL. Modifications of the water-insoluble humans lens α-crystallins. Exp Eye Res. 1996;63(6):661-672.

[14] Pintor J. Sugars, the Crystalline Lens and the Development of Cataracts. Biochem Pharmacol Open Access. 2012;01(04):10-12.

[15] Sorokanich S. Microscopic Findings .— The speci ¬ Martin Wand , MD. 2015;2015.

[16] Pollreisz A, Schmidt-Erfurth U. Diabetic Cataract—Pathogenesis, Epidemiology and Treatment. J Ophthalmol. 2010;2010:1-8.

[17] Kumar CM, Seet E, Eke T, Dhatariya K, Joshi GP. Glycaemic control during cataract surgery under loco-regional anaesthesia: a growing problem and we are none the wiser. Br J Anaesth. 2016;117(6):687-691.

[18] Onakpoya OH, Bekibele CO, Adegbehingbe SA. Control Study. 2009;16(2):88-92.

[19] Balasopoulou A, Kokkinos P, Pagoulatos D, Plotas P, Makri OE, Georgakopoulos CD, et al. Symposium Recent advances and challenges in the management of retinoblastoma

Globe - saving Treatments. BMC Ophthalmol. 2017;17(1):1.

[20] Okamoto F, Sone H, Nonoyama T, Hommura S. Refractive changes in diabetic patients during intensive glycaemic control. Br J Ophthalmol. 2000;84(10):1097-1102.

[21] Klein BEK, Lee KE, Klein R. Refraction in adults with diabetes. Arch Ophthalmol. 2011;129(1):56-62.

[22] Calvo-Maroto AM, Perez-Cambrodí RJ, Albarán-Diego C, Pons A, Cerviño A. Optical quality of the diabetic eye: A review. Eye. 2014;28(11):1271-1280.

[23] Kaštelan S, Gverović-Antunica A, Pelčić G, Gotovac M, Marković I, Kasun B. Refractive Changes Associated with Diabetes Mellitus. Semin Ophthalmol. 2018;33(7-8): 838-845.

[24] Jacobsen N, Jensen H, Lund-Andersen H, Goldschmidt E. Is poor glycaemic control in diabetic patients a risk factor of myopia? Acta Ophthalmol. 2008;86(5):510-514.

[25] Robinson et al. City Research Online City , University of London Institutional Repository. City Res Online. 2008;37(9):1591-1601.

[26] Neil Charman W, Atchison DA. Gradients of refractive index in the crystalline lens and transient changes in refraction among patients with diabetes. Biomed Opt Express. 2012;3(12):3033-30342.

[27] Neil Charman W, Atchison DA. Gradients of refractive index in the crystalline lens and transient changes in refraction among patients with diabetes. Biomed Opt Express. 2012;3(12):3033-3042.

[28] Valley SF, Bachelor H, Degree S, Therapy V, Ca P, Therapy V. Diabetes and Visual Dysfunction (OTHER) Pre - VT Progress Eval. 2016;

[29] Bron AJ, Sparrow J, Brown NAP, Harding JJ, Blakytny R. The lens in diabetes. Eye. 1993;7(2):260-275.

[30] Shih KC, Lam KL, Tong L. A systematic review on the impact of diabetes mellitus on the ocular surface. Nutr Diabetes. 2017;7(3):e251–e210.

[31] DelMonte DW, Kim T. Anatomy and physiology of the cornea. J Cataract Refract Surg. 2011;37(3):588-598.

[32] Ljubimov A V. Diabetic complications in the cornea. Vision Res. 2017;139:138-152.

[33] Wang B, Yang S, Zhai HL, Zhang YY, Cui CX, Wang JY, et al. A comparative study of risk factors for corneal infection in diabetic and non-diabetic patients. Int J Ophthalmol. 2018;11(1):43-47.

[34] Owen CG, Newsom RSB, Rudnicka AR, Barman SA, Woodward EG, Ellis TJ. Diabetes and the Tortuosity of Vessels of the Bulbar Conjunctiva. Ophthalmology. 2008;115(6):27-32.

[35] Achtsidis V, Eleftheriadou I, Kozanidou E, Voumvourakis KI, Stamboulis E, Theodosiadis PG, et al. Dry eye syndrome in subjects with diabetes and association with neuropathy. Diabetes Care. 2014;37(10):e210–e211.

[36] Zhang X, Zhao L, Deng S, Sun X, Wang N. Dry Eye Syndrome in Patients with Diabetes Mellitus: Prevalence, Etiology, and Clinical Characteristics. J Ophthalmol. 2016;2016:1-7.

[37] Voutilainen-Kaunisto R, Niskanen L, Uusitupa M, Teräsvirta M. Iris transluminance in type 2 diabetes. Acta Ophthalmol Scand. 2002;80(1):64-68.

[38] Wiley HE, Ferris FL. Nonproliferative Diabetic Retinopathy and Diabetic Macular Edema. Fifth Edit. Vol. 2, Retina Fifth Edition. Elsevier Inc.; 2012. 940-968 p.

[39] Ciulla TA, Amador AG, Zinman B. Diabetic retinopathy and diabetic macular edema: Pathophysiology, screening, and novel therapies. Diabetes Care. 2003;26(9):2653-2664.

[40] Vieira-Potter VJ, Karamichos D, Lee DJ. Ocular Complications of Diabetes and Therapeutic Approaches. Biomed Res Int. 2016;2016.

[41] Howells LH. Ocular complications of diabetes mellitus. Br J Ophthalmol. 1953;37(12):716-724.

[42] Qian H, Ripps H. Neurovascular interaction and the pathophysiology of diabetic retinopathy. Exp Diabetes Res. 2011;2011.

[43] Negi A, Vernon SA. An overview of the eye in diabetes. J R Soc Med. 2003;96(6):266-272.

[44] Brownlee M, Aiello LP, Cooper ME, Vinik AI, Plutzky J, Boulton AJM. Complications of Diabetes Mellitus BIOCHEMISTRY AND MOLECULAR CELL BIOLOGY. Thirteenth. Biochemistry and Molecular Cell Biology. Elsevier Inc.; 2017. 1484-1581 p.

[45] Su RF, Su C, Tan XB, Zhang L. Effect of panretinal photocoagulation on retinal nerve fiber layer thickness and visual field in diabetic retinopathy. Int Eye Sci. 2020;20(1):154-157.

[46] Khan A, Petropoulos IN, Ponirakis G, Malik RA. Visual complications in diabetes mellitus: beyond retinopathy. Diabet Med. 2017;34(4):478-484.

[47] Jabs DA, Miller NR, Green WR. Ischaemic optic neuropathy with painful ophthalmoplegia in diabetes mellitus. 1981;673-678.

[48] Al Kahtani ES, Khandekar R, Al-Rubeaan K, Youssef AM, Ibrahim HM, Al-Sharqawi AH. Assessment of the prevalence and risk factors of ophthalmoplegia among diabetic patients in a large national diabetes registry cohort. BMC Ophthalmol. 2016;16(1):1-8.

[49] Shrestha GS, Kaiti R. Visual functions and disability in diabetic retinopathy patients. J Optom. 2014;7(1):37-43.

[50] Tan NC, Yip WF, Kallakuri S, Sankari U, Koh YLE. Factors associated with impaired color vision without retinopathy amongst people with type 2 diabetes mellitus: A cross-sectional study. BMC Endocr Disord. 2017;17(1):1-8.

[51] Di Leo MAS, Caputo S, Falsini B, Porciatti V, Minnella A, Greco A V., et al. Nonselective loss of contrast sensitivity in visual system testing in early type I diabetes. Diabetes Care. 1992;15(5):620-625.

[52] Verrotti A, Lobefalo L, Petitti MT, Mastropasqua L, Morgese G, Chiarelli F, et al. Relationship between contrast sensitivity and metabolic control in diabetics with and without retinopathy Relationship between contrast sensitivity and metabolic control in diabetics with and without retinopathy. 2009;3890.

[53] Safi S, Rahimi A, Raeesi A, Safi H, Amiri MA, Malek M, et al. Contrast sensitivity to spatial gratings in moderate and dim light conditions in patients with diabetes in the absence of diabetic retinopathy. 2017;1-9.

[54] Lavin PJM. hemianopia : A reversible complication of non-ketotic hyperglycemia. Neurology. 2005;65:616-619.

[55] Fors M. Some Considerations about Glucose Determination in Humor Vitreous to Estimate Post Mortem Interval. Curr Res Diabetes Obes J. 2018;7(4):3-5.

[56] Mhatre V. Ho and Kelsey C. Martin J-AL. Acute Hypoglycemia Decreases Central Retinal Function in the Human Eye. Bone. 2012;23(1):1-7.

[57] Sharma T, Kaur H, Weinstock RS. Visual Symptoms During Hypoglycemia: A Case Series. AACE Clin Case Reports. 2015;1(1):e32–e35.

Chapter 4

Biological Responses to the Consumption of Non-Nutritional Sweeteners

Sage Arbor

Abstract

Non-nutritive sweetener (NNS) use has increased exponentially over the last 30 years as industrialized countries attempted, and failed, to battle obesity epidemics. Large studies have now shown that consumption of NNS's does not help obese individuals lose weight. A large number of scientific studies on NNS's effects have many conflicting results, methodological issues, conflicts of interest, while double blind studies represent a small minority of the studies. NNS's have often been considered as a group despite having unique in vivo absorption, distribution, metabolism, and excretion (ADME). Aspartame may be the most desirable NNS due to its rapid degradation in vivo, whereas saccharin and sucralose are worrisome due to their extended stability in vivo. This review will focus on the most ubiquitous NNS's: aspartame, saccharin, acesulfame-K, sucralose, stevia, sugar alcohols (sorbitol, xylitol, and erythritol), and discuss their different chemical structures, metabolism, effect on the gut biome and cancer.

Keywords: artificial sweetener, sweet receptor, gut brain axis, obesity, diet

1. Introduction

Non-nutritive sweeteners (NNS's) contain few to no calories or nutrients. As obesity had been rising in western countries at the end of the 20th century, NNS use increased 54% in adults and a staggering 200% in children from 2000 to 2010 [1, 2]. In 2018 over $7 billion (USD) NNS's (also called artificial sweeteners or sugar substitutes) were sold which is projected to grow 5%/year reaching more than $10 billion by 2025 [3]. However recent reports have shown NAS's to be ineffective at reducing obesity [4, 5], which is their primary health target. Malek et al. found that while consumers of NNS's reported lower caloric intake compared to non-NNS consumers, the NNS consumers were more overweight and obese [4]. While the "Calories in - Calories Out" (CICO) paradigm governing net weight gain/loss of has been resoundingly confirmed [6–8], the mechanism causing NAS's to be ineffective at reducing weight are still being investigated. Does NAS consumption cause increased appetite for food with caloric content (calories in)? Is metabolism and movement decreased (calories out)? Are effects mostly due to human cellular or gut microbiome response? How consistent are these effects across the NNS's, and lastly how individual are these effects? Genetic polymorphisms have been elucidated which do personalize an individual's experience to NAS's [9, 10], but this does not appear to be a primary driver since obesity has risen on a population and indeed global level.

The safety thresholds for human consumable substances are set by national or international organizations, and this review will highlight the work done by three organizations: the Joint Expert Committee on Food Additives (JECFA), European Union's Scientific Committee for Food (SCF), and the US Food and Drug Administration (FDA). Eight NNS's have been approved by the FDA: aspartame, acesulfame potassium, luo han guo (monk) fruit extract, neotame, saccharin, stevia, sucralose and advantame [11]. While this group, along with sugar alcohols, are often grouped as sugar replacements they differ in their in vivo stability, targets, and even caloric content to a minor extent. The differences between their structures, metabolism, effect on gut biome, host metabolism, obesity, cancer, and future human studies will be discussed.

2. Biological effects of artificial sweeteners

Non-nutritive sweeteners (NNS's) were designed to mimic the sweetness of sugar without containing any caloric content. However, over the last 40 years robust biological effects have been demonstrated beyond the desired sweetness profile. Artificial sweeteners differ in structure, in vivo half-life, molecular targets, effect on host gut-biome, and magnitude of biological effect. Consumer products increasingly have mixed NNS's to augment their flavor profile, which makes survey study results less useful since questions such as "how many diet sodas did you drink per week" can encompass biological responses from an unknown mix of NNS's. The specific attributes and effects for the major NSS's will be reviewed below.

2.1 Structure and metabolism of artificial sweeteners

While Non-nutritive sweeteners (NNS's) have a detectably different flavor profile [12, 13], they largely overlap in successfully replacing the sensation of sugar in foods and beverages. As a group NNS's are much more potent at stimulating the sensation of sweetness in the mouth compared to table sugar. There is concern that such swamping of one's taste receptors with sweetness through excessive NNS consumption could limit the desirability of more complex flavors, making less sweet food (e.g. fruit) less appealing, and causing healthy unsweet foods (e.g. vegetables) to be newly intolerable. NNS's differ in chemical structure by over 5-fold in molecular weight (MW) (**Table 1**). Saccharin is the lightest at 183 MW, while Rebaudioside A (a steviol glycoside) is a whopping 967 MW which causes stevias elimination (urine vs. feces) to differ between mammals based on billary excretion MW thresholds [17, 18]. The safety of NNS's are initially determined from taxoicokinetic studies in various animal models, such as mice and rats, which absorption, distribution, metabolism, and excretion (ADME) after ingestion. The animal model with results that most closely match the ADME characteristics seen during human consumption are used to set safety limits. A wide range of NNS concentrations are used so the high doses can elucidate any adverse effects, while the lower doses titrate these potential adverse effects away until the "no observed adverse effect level" (NOAEL) is determined. Adverse effects measured to determine NOAEL may include changes in development, morphology, growth, or lifespan. The NOAEL is used to determine the acceptable daily intake (ADI), which is usually set at 100 times lower than the NOAEL. Therefore, while the ADI is often misinterpreted as a "line in the sand", a level above which a compound is instantly toxic. However, in reality the ADI is a warning level that should be much lower than toxicity while allowing up to a two fold increase before deleterious effects are seen. A significant caveat to this paradigm for NNS's is that long term human changes in

Name	Saccharin	Sucralose	Aspartame	Stevioside	Acesulfame-K	Neotame	Advantame	Cyclamate	Sugar alcohols
Structure	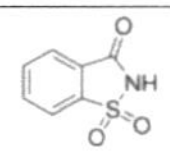	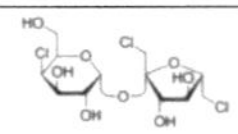	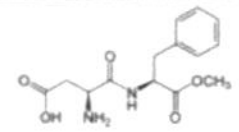	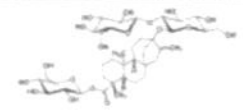	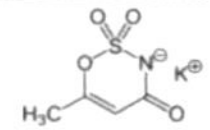	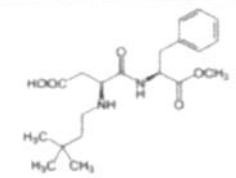	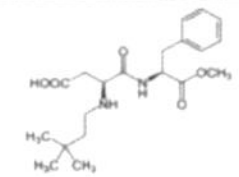	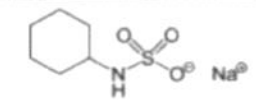	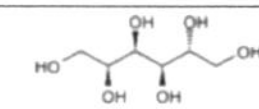
Molecular weight (g/mol)	183.18	397.6	294.3	804.87	201.2	378.5	458.5	201.22	122–182
Other names	Sweet and Low, Sweet Twin, Necta Sweet	Splenda, Zerocal, Sukrana, SucraPlus, Nevella	Nutrasweet, Equal, Sugar Twin	Stevia extract, rebaudioside A	Sunett, Ace K Sweet & Safe, SweetOne	Newtame	N/A	Sucaryl, Sugar Twin	Sorbitol, Xylitol, Erythritol
Sweetness compared to 10% sucrose solution	300×	600×	200×	30-320×	200×	7000–13,000×	20,000×	30-50×	0.7×
pKa	1.6	12.5	3.1, 7.9	11.8	2.0	3.0, 8.1	2.9, 8.0	1.7	13
Year discovered	1879	1976	1965	1931	1967	FDA approved (US)	FDA approved (US) 2014	1937	1920
Nutritional calories/g	0	0	4	0	0	0	0	0	2.4
Bind receptors outside of oral cavity [10, 14, 15]	T2R8, T2R43, T2R31	t1R3	None	T2R4, T2R14	T2R9, T2R43, T2R31	No	No	T2R1, T2R31, T2R38 T2R43	T1R2, T1R3
Absorption in humans unmodified (modified)	85%	15%	0%, (100% as digested products)	0% steviol glycoside, (100% (steviol)	100%	34%	6%	50%	50%

Name	Saccharin	Sucralose	Aspartame	Stevioside	Acesulfame-K	Neotame	Advantame	Cyclamate	Sugar alcohols
Main site of metabolism	None	None	GI tract	Liver	None	Entire body	None	Gut biome	Liver
ADI (mg/kg/day)	15	5	50	4	15	0.3	33	11	N/A
*ADI (# Sweetener Packets Equivalent) [16]	45	23	75	9	23	23	4920	N/A	N/A
**ADI (# 12 oz. sodas Equivalent)	10	5	16	?	20	?	?	?	?

ADI = Accepted Daily Value.
**Number of Tabletop Sweetener Packets a 60 kg (132 pound) person would need to consume to reach the ADI. Calculations assume a packet of high-intensity sweetener is as sweet as two teaspoons of sugar. Adapted from: Kim Y, Keogh JB, Clifton PM. Non-nutritive Sweeteners and Glycaemic Control. Curr Atheroscler Rep. 2019 19;21(12):49. [16]*
***ADI (# 12 oz. sodas) was calculated for a 60 kg person, using the following brands and concentrations: 90 mg saccharin in Tab; 60 mg sucralose in Diet Coke with Splenda; 187 mg aspartame in Diet Coke; 45 mg acesulfame-K in Diet Coke with Splenda. Note splenda and acesulfame-K are mixed in multiple diet beverages such as Diet Coke with Splenda shown in this table.*
? The mg of NNS could not be found for commercially sold drinks with stevioside, neotame, advantame, cyclacate, sugar alcohols.

Table 1.
Comparison of non-nutritive sweetener characteristics.

caloric balance, such as increased caloric consumption due to unbalanced sweetness perception, would likely not be discovered in an initial NOAEL study.

There are synthetic sweeteners (acesulfame K, aspartame, cyclamate, saccharin, neotame, advantame, and sucralose), natural sweeteners (thaumatin, steviol glucosides, monellin, neohesperidin dihydrochalcone, and glycyrrhizin), and nutritive sweeteners (polyols or sugar alcohols). In 2017 the world consumed 159,000 metric tons of NNS's (valued at $2 billion USD). China was the top region consuming NNS's (32%) followed by Asia/Oceania (23%), United States (23%), Europe (12%), and then Africa (7%) [19]. The NNS most used in food and drink was aspartame, followed by saccharin, acesulfame, and sucralose (18.5, 9.7, 6.8, and 3.3 thousand metric tons respectively) [20]. With the quantities of NNS being produced and consumed both increasing rapidly, their contamination in the environment has been of concern [21]. There has been quantitative reports finding NNS's in surface water (e.g. lakes, rivers, streams), groundwater, tap water, discharge into the sea, and even in the atmosphere [22], as well as passing through Waste Water Treatment Plants (WWTPs) [23]. NNS's have been found to interfere with photosynthesis, creating disturbances in carbon dioxide intake [24], and decreasing sugar breakdown in human body [25, 26]. The exposure to any of these environmental NNS's would likely be orders of magnitude lower than current self-selected consumption levels. Acesulfame-potassium (Ace-K) was investigated, as an environmentally persistent NNS due to low biodegradation, and found to not pose an environmental risk with very low levels in surface water and even less in groundwater (lower parts per billion [ppb] range and lower parts per trillion [ppt] respectively) [27].

The metabolism of the main NNS's can largely be put into 3 bins [28]: aspartame which is broken up when it hits the GI tract, artificial sweeteners that enter the GI tract (stevia, cyclamate, sucralose, acesulfame potassium), and sugar alcohols which can contribute calories to the diet. Cyclamate is not used in the US, and not widely used in Canada due to concerns about carcinogenesis. Advantame and neotame being newer compounds to the market also do not represent a large portion of the market.

2.1.1 Aspartame

Aspartame is 200 times sweeter than sugar, the most ubiquitous of the NNS's, and is quickly digested into aspartic acid, phenylalanine, and methanol. Due to its amino acid constituency aspartame is strictly a nutritive sweetener. However, because 100 g of sugar can be replaced by less than a gram of aspartame, it is consumed in such low levels that it is considered as a NNS [29]. The phenylalanine can build up to toxic levels in those with a rare genetic defect, phenylketonuria (PKU) present for 1 in 12,000 births [30], caused by mutations and lower levels in the enzyme phenylalanine hydroxylase (PAH). Infants are diagnosed with PKU shortly after birth and avoiding aspartame is achieved well by patients throughout life [31]. However, people with PKU do show increased oxidative stress [32] and the presence of comorbidities including asthma, alopecia, urticaria, gallbladder disease, rhinitis, esophageal disorders, anemia, overweight, GERD, eczema, renal insufficiency, osteoporosis, gastritis/esophagitis and kidney stones [33]. Methanol, which is converted to formaldehyde (a known carcinogen) [34], is often pointed to as a reason to avoid aspartame, but higher levels of methanol are consumed when eating fruit [35, 36]. The FDA set the ADI of aspartame at 50 mg/kg/day and, despite consumption increases since the 1980s, the US average and 95th percentile intake in 2013 was 4.9 and 13.3 mg/kg/day respectively, showing consumption levels are still 4 fold below the ADI. While some customers have complained of an aspartame sensitivity a double blind study found there to be no evidence of any acute adverse response [37]. Aspartame holds a unique position among NNS's in that its pharmacophore structure which binds sweet receptors is obliterated by esterases and peptidases shortly after consumption when it enters the gastrointestinal (GI) tract. Many of the NNS's have been shown to bind sweet receptors outside of the oral cavity, such as in the digestive tract. Among all the NNS's consumers can be most confident that aspartame will not elicit endogenous sweet receptor cascades after swallowing due to its rapid degradation early in the GI tract (**Figure 1**).

2.1.2 Saccharin

Saccharin was one of the leading NNS's used during the early increase in global consumption (along with aspartame), but lost market share in the 1980s due to a 1978 paper suggesting rats had an increase in carcinomas in their urinary bladder upon exposure [38]. Since then studies have shown saccharin does not cause urinary cancer in humans and the carcinoma in mice may have been due to the large amounts of sodium administered (as sodium saccharin) [39]. Saccharin has a pKa of 1.8 and is absorbed better in species with a low stomach pH (e.g. rabbits and humans compared to the higher pH in rats). Being very water soluble there is no build up of saccharin in tissues. In humans ~90% is absorbed and excreted

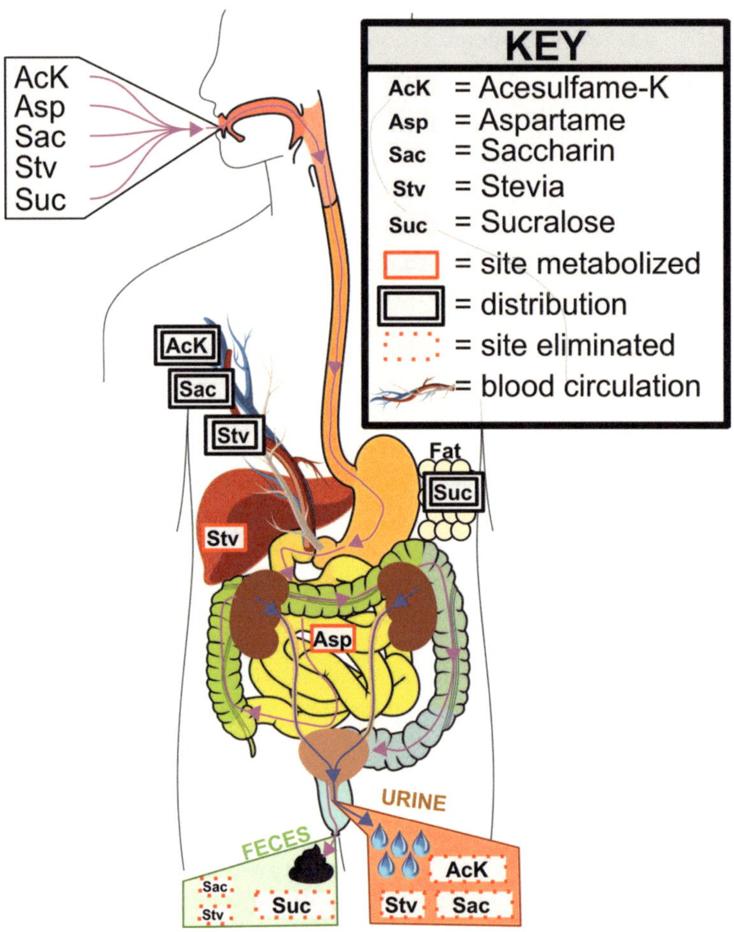

Figure 1.
Metabolism and excretion of non-nutritive sweeteners. NNS's differ in their in vivo stability, distribution, and excretion. Acesulfame-K, saccharin, stevia enter the bloodstream and are mostly excreted in the urine. Sucralose exists via the feces but can accumulate in fat when in an acetylated form. Red box: Site of metabolism where NSS is degraded. Black double box: Site of distribution or accumulation. Dashed red box: Site of elimination.

in the urine while only ~10% exits in the feces. Discovered in 1878, saccharins use started to increase around 1900 when it was initially used as a sweetener by diabetic patients, but during the world wars its use in food increased because there were sugar shortages [40]. The stability of saccharin decreases above 125°C which diminishes its usefulness in cooking [40]. Saccharin is 300-fold sweeter than sugar, 1.5-fold sweeter than aspartame, and even among heavy consumers (~2 mg/kg/day) [41, 42] its usage levels are below the ADI of 5 mg/kg/day [43]. While saccharin requires less of a dose than aspartame to attain the same sweetness, it does have an undesirable metallic taste at high concentrations [44]. Saccharin can cross the placental barrier in rats, monkeys, and humans with maternal tissues having higher steady-state levels than the fetus, though the concentration in the fetal tissue does decrease slower than in maternal tissues. Therefore, mothers do not need to be as concerned with saccharin building up in their fetus, but if lowering consumption there will be a delay in lowering levels in the fetus. Of note, while saccharin buildup itself may not be an issue for the fetus, the effect of NNS's on the maternal metabolism can have knock-on effects which do seem to affect the fetus. Consistent NNS consumption is associated with glucose intolerance, interference with energy homeostasis [45–47], and if occurring during pregnancy is associated with increased chances of obesity for the child after birth [46–48].

2.1.3 Acesulfame-K

Acesulfame potassium (Ace-K) is a non-nutritive sweetener discovered in 1967 when a researcher accidentally tasted a new synthesis compound. Often labeled as one of the more pleasant tasting NNS's (no metallic taste), Ace-K is commercially attractive due to its 200-fold greater sweetness than sugar, along with excellent solubility and stability in water [49, 50]. Multiple organizations (JECFA in 1983, SCF in 1985, and the FDA in 1988), agreed that there were no adverse effects in either rats or dogs over a 2-year period when fed up to 3% Ace-K [43]. Using the body weights this led to NOAELs of 900 and 1500 mg/kg/day for dogs and rats respectively. The JECFA and FDA used the rat study to set the ADI at 15 mg/kg/day while SCF used the dog study to set the ADI at 9 mg/kg/day [51]. Ace-K is not metabolized in humans, but can degrade into acetoacetamide. Radiolabeling studies showing intact Ace-K (and zero breakdown products) in serum, urine, feces and/or bile [43, 50, 51]. In humans 98% of a 30 mg Ace-K dose was excreted in urine within 24 hours. In pregnant women 1.6% of radiolabeled Ace-K was excreted in milk in 24 hours, which dropped by an order of magnitude the next day (to 0.16%). The highest Ace-K concentration (0.4 mg/kg) occurred in humans 1.5 hours after consumption [52].

2.1.4 Sucralose

Recently a study in rats has shown that sucralose (80 mg/kg/day for 40 days) converted to acetylated forms of sucralose, which are less polar, deposit in fat tissue due to their lipophilicity (**Figure 1**). These acetylated sucralose compounds were detected 6 days after unmodified sucralose had left the body. The original studies and regulatory decision process were unaware of these metabolites or accumulation in adipose tissue due to use of a methanol fraction from feces for analysis [27]. Sucralose is a chlorinated carbohydrate, which has been found to persistently exist in wastewater treatment plant effluents and downstream aquatic environments. Free chlorine, ozone, and ferrate did not degrade sucralose in water, but strong oxidizing agent hydroxyl radicals (•OH) was able to degrade sucralose in water [53].

In animal and human studies sucralose has been shown to not have carcinogenic activity, even when consumed at doses several orders of magnitude more than normal consumption levels [54]. Sucralose largely passes through the digestive tract and is eliminated in feces unchanged (85%) [54]. The remaining 15% of sucralose does distribute throughout the body, but because there is not active transport there are not significant levels in breast milk or across the blood–brain barrier into the central nervous system. There is 2–3% of consumed sucralose undergoing phase II metabolism (glucuronidation) and, along with the other 12% that was initially retained, is excreted in the urine [55–57].

2.1.5 Stevia

Stevia is not absorbed, whereas cyclamate and sucralose are partially absorbed but still not metabolized. Steviol glycosides and luo han guo fruit extracts are categorized as natural sweeteners by the FDA and therefore regulated differently [58]. Steviol glycosides are actually a group of compounds which are metabolized differently with varying biological effects, and while usually derived from the *Stevia rebaudiana* Bertoni plant, can also be produced via fermentation [59]. All steviol glycosides share a common chemical core structure, diterpene steviol (the final product of colonic bacterial metabolism). The Joint Expert Committee on Food Additives (JECFA) established an upper acceptable daily intake (ADI) of 2 mg/kg/day based on the amount of steviol after digestion which has been termed the "steviol equivalent". For example, 3 mg of rebaudioside A converts to just 1 mg of steviol equivalent. Steviol glycosides are not metabolized in the upper gastrointestinal tract, but once reaching the colon bacteria convert them to steviol compounds which travel to the liver and are glucuronidated to steviol glucuronide [24] (**Figure 1**). Increasing levels of steviol glucuronide can be detected to peak in the plasma in humans 8 hours after administration, with a half-life of ~14 hours. In rats almost all of radiolabeled steviol glycosides were found in feces, with less than 2% showing up in urine [25]. However in humans steviol glucuronide was excreted in urine not feces, due to a difference in biliary excretion molecular weight thresholds compared to rats [17, 18]. The glucose that is removed from the glycosides in the colon is not absorbed as caloric input by humans, and is assumed to be quickly consumed by the colonic bacteria.

2.1.6 Sugar alcohols (sorbitol, xylitol, and erythritol)

While sugar alcohols (sorbitol, xylitol, and erythritol) are often binned with all of the sugar substitutes, they are not actually NNS's since they do contribute usable calories for humans. Sorbitol, xylitol, and erythritol are carbon chains with an alcohol attached to each carbon and differ structurally only in their carbon length with 6, 5, and 4 carbons respectively (**Table 1**). Sorbitol has low absorption, is hyperosmotic causing laxative effects, and is metabolized to fructose (via sorbitol dehydrogenase). Xylitol has low absorption in the GI tract, and is processed in the pentose phosphate pathway (PPP). Erythritol is absorbed but not metabolized and has negligible calories compared to sorbitol or xylitol. Generally the NNS's do not increase blood glucose levels with an exception being xylitol and maltitol which increase blood glucose about 40% and 80% as much as sugar respectively [24].

2.2 Effect on gut biome

The human body has been estimated to have 10-fold more bacterial symbiotic cells than human cells. The gut microbiome contains 10^{14} microorganisms that play a role in host nutrition, proliferation of intestinal cells, bone mineralization, xenobiotic metabolism, immune system regulation and protection against pathogens [60]. The effect of NAS of gut microbiome is clearly augmented by multiple NAS and could be responsible for a significant fraction of the negative population level obesity increases. In an elegant paper Suez et al. showed NAS consumption led to glucose intolerance through induction of compositional and functional alterations to the intestinal microbiota [61]. Mice fed saccharin, sucralose, or aspartame all showed increased blood glucose during an oral glucose test (>250 mg/dl at 15 min. Vs 200 mg/dl for sucrose or glucose), as well as increased area under the two-hour blood glucose response curve (AUC) after 11 weeks of consuming NAS. These deleterious effects were abrogated by antibiotic treatment, but were fully transferrable to germ-free mice upon fecal transplantation of microbiota configurations from NAS-consuming mice. Saccharin exhibited the greatest glucose intolerance and was further studied. Interestingly mice fed saccharin did not show differences in liquid or chow consumption, oxygen consumption, walking distance or energy expenditure. In contrast the gut microbiome of the mice fed saccharin did change significantly, with more than 40 operational taxonomic units (OTUs) significantly altered in abundance. Taxa that increased in relative abundance belonged to the Bacteroides genus and Clostridiales order, while other members of the Clostridiales order comprised the majority of under-represented taxa, along with Lactobacillus reuteri, with similar effects in germ-free recipients of stools from saccharin-consuming donors [61]. A similar NAS-induced dysbiosis and glucose intolerance was demonstrated in healthy human subjects (based on a validated food frequency questionnaire) [61]. However Ruiz-Ojeda et al. (2019) reviewed the NNS's and found only sucralose, saccharin, and stevia to have evidence of effecting the gut microbiota. Sucralose could cause dysbiosis by lowering the total number of bifidobacteria, lactobacilli, Bacteriodes, and Clostridiales (both aerobic and anaerobic species) [62]. A study in 2017 found sucralose could increase Clostridium cluster XIVa in mice [63]. A positive correlation was found between NAS consumption and multiple metabolic-syndrome-related clinical parameters including: increased weight and waist-to-hip ratio (measures of central obesity), higher fasting blood glucose, glycosylated hemoglobin (HbA1C% indicative of glucose concentration over the previous 3 months) and glucose tolerance test (GTT, measures of impaired glucose tolerance). A small study was also done following seven healthy non-NAS consuming volunteers for 1 week (5 males and 2 females, aged 28–36) in which they consumed the FDA's maximal acceptable daily intake (ADI) of commercial saccharin (5 mg/kg body weight, as 120 mg x 3times/day) and were monitored by continuous glucose measurements and daily GTT. Even in the short 7-day exposure period, most individuals (4 out of 7) developed significantly poorer glycaemic responses [61].

Consuming larger amounts of non-caloric artificial sweeteners (NAS) have been found to increase in hemoglobin (HbA1C %), as well as increased levels of Enterobacteriaceae family, Deltaproteobacteria class, and Actinobacteria phylum found in fecal microbiota [61]. There have been literature reviews that found such effects to be inconsistent with methodological or reporting problems concluding that NAS's (e.g., acesulfame K, aspartame, cyclamate, neotame, saccharin, sucralose, steviol glycosides) have no evidence of an actual adverse effect on human health [64]. Such reviews often point out that studies showing changes in the diet unrelated to NAS consumption may be confounding the data. It is worth noting that such studies can be funded by corporate entities with conflicts of interest, such as the Calorie Control Council (established in 1966 as an international association representing the low- and reduced-calorie food and beverage industry) [64]. A 2016 systematic study on risk of bias screened 493 papers publishing about NNS and, after analyzing the 31 papers that met the eligibility requirements, found extremely statistically significant bias [65]. Reviews that were sponsored by the artificial sweetener industry were 1700% more likely to have favorable results (Relative Risk (RR) = 17.25). Not only do industry reported papers supporting the use of NNS's seem unreliable, but all 4 papers analyzed that were funded by NNS competitor companies (sugar and water industry) found unfavorable conclusions. A disturbing 42% of reviews did not have authors' financial conflicts of interest disclosed. Lastly reviews performed by authors with financial conflicts of interest almost always had favorable conclusions (18/22, RR = 7.36) [65].

Aspartame and acesulfame-K have been found to not interact with the human colonic microbiota, whereas saccharin and sucralose change the gut microbiome populations (though those effects are not clearly positive or detrimental) [66]. Sugar alcohols can also reach the colonic microbiota and act as prebiotics, with accompanying negative laxative effects [67], particularly in patients with inflammatory bowel syndrome (IBS). Since sucralose can deposit in fat tissue in an acelatyed version (see metabolism section), studies that have looked at the effect of sucralose with less than a week washout period could have to be revisited [68].

While most studies have just measured disturbances or lack thereof from NNS's there have been some advancements in the physiological and mechanistic effects gut microbiome dysbiosis could cause. One leading concern would be if NNS's can lead t0 Non-alcoholic fatty liver disease (NAFLD). NAFLD is denoted by an excess fat in the liver in people who do not drink significant alcohol. Gut dysbiosis has a continually increasing number of known effects including altering caloric absorption [69], development of a "leaky gut", increase in bile acid receptors and transporters, as well as choline deficiency. A leaky gut allows proinflammatory molecules and bacterial endotoxins (e.g. LPS and ethanol) to enter the bloodstream, travel through the portal vein to the liver and increase hepatic inflammation which leads to NAFLD. Increases in bile acid lead to insulin resistance and NAFLD [60]. Dysbiosis in the gut increases conversion of choline to dimethylamine (DMA) and trimethylamine (TMA) [70, 71], potentially leading to choline deficiency which decreases the transportation of VLDL which is used to mobilize fat from the liver [60].

2.3 Effect on host metabolism and obesity

Glucose (which NSS's mimic) has long been known as the in vivo "nutrient sensor", not only for carbohydrates consumed but as a "fed state" signal in general since muscular protein can be broken down to produce glucose (via gluconeogenesis). However it appears that the dose dependent glucose detection of sweetness, which matches the caloric load of that glucose, is also an important input for our in vivo nutrient sensor. Recent evidence suggests NNS consumption disrupts our normal association if sweetness levels detected differ from caloric intake, causing us to crave even more sweets and gain weight. Indeed, the San Antonio Heart Study found those who drank more than 21 diet drinks per week were found to be twice as likely to become overweight or obese as people who did not drink diet soda [72].

2.3.1 Sweetness and caloric load alignment for maximal metabolic response

A ground breaking study by Veldhuizen et al. found that for carbohydrate reward to maximize its biological response the level of sweet taste must match the caloric load that natural carbohydrate food would provide [73]. The level of caloric load was manipulated using maltodextrin, a tasteless carbohydrate, while the sweetness levels were manipulated with the NNS sucralose. Beverages with differing amounts of maltodextrin + sucralose showed a non-linear response between caloric load, metabolic response and reinforcement potency. When sweetness is proportional to caloric load greater metabolic responses are observed. Lower calorie beverages were able to produce greater metabolic response than a beverage with more calories but the same level of sweetness, and that data was integrated in the Central Nervous System (CNS). fMRI studies showed the nucleus accumbens (NAcc) response was also greatest when sweetness and caloric load were balanced [73]. It understandably appears humans have evolved to elicit a maximum metabolic response to carbohydrate when the caloric load matches the sweetness that natural sugars such as glucose induce. The use of NNS's are almost always used to replace the sweetness lost when calories are removed from processed foods or beverages, which is now know to elicit a submaximal metabolic response.

2.3.2 Nutrient sensing

Approximately 1% of the mucosal epithelial layer of the gastrointestinal (GI) tract are made up of hormone-secreting enteroendocrine (EE) cells, which by mass are the largest endocrine tissue in the body. It is now understood that whole-body metabolism integrates signals from many metabolically active tissues (GI tract, pancreas, adipose tissue, liver, and the CNS). These organs can release both nutrient storage hormones in the fed state postprandially (e.g. glucagon-like peptide-1 (GLP-1), gastric inhibitory peptide (GIP, also known as: glucose-dependent insulinotropic polypeptide), peptide tyrosine tyrosine (PYY), Cholecystokinin (CCK), Oxyntomodulin (OXM)) or after a period of fasting (e.g. ghrelin, 5-hydroxytryptamine (5-HT, also known as gut-derived serotonin when released by the intestine)). Agonists of the sweet taste receptors in the GI tract modifies secretion of GLP-1, PYY, ghrelin, and GIP which appears to increase the storage of blood glucose [5] (to glycogen or triacylglycerides and preferential differentiation into adipocytes) [58]. Glucose causes GLP-1 secretion via glucose-dependent Na^+ uptake via SGLT-1 and intracellular glucose metabolism, closing the KATP channels, causing further depolarisation and exocytosis [74]. The distal portion of the small intestine in particular regulates glucose uptake via release of incretins (GLP-1, GIP) [74]. While many of these hormonal links to metabolic syndrome have been elucidated, such as increased 5-HT gut-derived serotonin levels in type II diabetics, most of the knowledge covers the correlation of hormone levels with disease and the downstream effects (such as increased lipogenisis) but not the breadth and magnitude of molecular mechanisms causing this. For example, while serotonin is most often thought of for its neurotransmitter effects in the CNS, more than 90% of whole body 5-HT levels are produced in enterochromaffin (EC) cells in the intestinal epithelium lining and platlets. These EC cells in the gut lumen detect multiple nutritional moieties such as glucose and fructose [75, 76], medium chain fatty acids, as well as various tastants and olfactants [77]. Studies of such EC cell stimulation are confounded by the fact that they are also regulated by mechanical stimulation, neural and endocrine inputs (e.g. adrenergic stimulation and GABA and somatostatin inhibition) [78]. The increased gut-derived 5-HT during a fasted state, along with glucagon, increases hepatic gluconeogenesis and glycogenolysis and therefore glucose output from the liver, while also inhibiting glucose uptake or glycogen synthesis at the liver. At the same time 5-HT increases lypolysis in white fat cells.

Under fasting conditions, gut-derived 5-HT, together with glucagon, markedly increases hepatic glucose output, a main driver of fasting euglycaemia, by increasing hepatic gluconeogenesis and glycogenolysis (29), while inhibiting glucose uptake and glycogen synthesis in the liver (30). 5-HT promotes not only lipolysis, but also energy conservation and weight gain via reduced thermogenesis in brown adipose tissue (and hence reduced energy expenditure) [79]. Antagonists and agonists of these caloric receptors, such as NNS's, have to be considered in the hormone secretion per cell. However as an example, HT-5 also increases the density or glucose-sensitivity of duodenal EC cells, which can be measured in obese human duodenal EC cells [80], but the molecular mechanisms producing this increased density have not been elucidated.

Because adipocytes (both undifferentiated and mature) express sweet and bitter taste receptors [69], a direct role of NNS's in adipocyte differentiation and function is likely. Both acesulfame-K and saccharin bind the bitter taste receptors at higher concentrations adding the complexity of a second pathway they stimulate compared to many other NNS's [70]. Sucralose was found to promote fat accumulation and upregulate adipogenesis, inflammation, and antioxidant pathways [71]. While rodents lacking sweet taste receptor subunits were shown to have less adiposity and smaller adipocytes on a Western diet [32], showing the importance of sweet taste receptor signaling for normal adipose tissue development. One study suggested NNS's were not dependent on sweet taste receptors to stimulate adipogenesis or suppress lipolysis [36]. However in contrast, Masubuchi et al. reported that adipogenesis was inhibited by sucralose and saccharin in preadipocytes [72], and suggested NNS exposure leads to microtubule disassembly and alteration of the PI3K–Akt signaling pathway [72]. The rodent and in vitro studies do not provide conclusive results [58].

A pattern has emerged in which observational studies make NNS's appear harmful causing increased weight, while intervention studies find NNS's reduce weight. A natural hypothesis was that in the observational studies the people consuming NNS's must have compensated by eating more solid food calories at subsequent meals, which indeed was found in some studies, but others reported a reduction in total energy expenditure after NNS consumption [81]. When sweet receptors in the oral cavity are activated not only does the brain perceive sweetness but the body prepares to digest calories through the cephalic phase responses, most notably the cephalic phase insulin response (CPIR) which is a neurally-mediated release of insulin prior to nutrient absorption [82]. Not only do glucose [83] and sucrose [82] stimulate CPIR, but saccharin [82] and possibly sucralose [84] also to activate CPIR. Of note, all these molecules which activate CPIR seem to bind the same VFD region on the T1R3 receptor [84]. In contrast aspartame [84, 85], stevioside and cyclamate [86] all bind a different site on the receptor and fail to elicit the CPIR response. If this CPIR were the main driver of obesity and driven by binding the VFD region on T1R3 then those consuming saccharin and sucralose would be expected to have increased Total Body Weight (TBW) compared to those consume aspartate, stevioside, or cyclamate. However, that has been neither proven nor disproven. In addition while CPIR may be activated through the sweet receptor recent studies have suggested that CPIR may actually be activated through the adenosine triphosphate (ATP)-sensitive potassium channel (K_{ATP} channels) [87] which are also found on T1R3-containing taste cells [88].

The magnitude with which the combination of circadian rhythm and eating controls metabolism at a cellular level is currently a productive field of research. The use of NSS's during fasting would be useful to not only elucidate the pathways augmented by NNS's while removing confounding variables, but would also shed some needed information on to what degree, if any, NNS's inhibit the positive molecular effects of fasting. It is now well documented that extended fasts (> = 1 day) increase autophagy (recycling of cellular content) [89–93] which has been shown to be anti-cancer [94], anti-aging [93, 95–100], beneficial to sleep [101–103], protective of muscle loss [89, 104], and clearly helpful to reduce weight [105–109]. Many people that undergo intermittent fasting still consume diet beverages because they are viewed as low or zero calorie. Quality-Adjusted Life Years (QALYs) analyses for NNS's, incorporating data across multiple disease states, would be useful in determining the utility of NSS's (e.g. positive tastant stimulant vs. negative microbiome modulator). The main QALY studies found in pubmed by the author concerned the efficacy of sugar taxes to increase QALYs [110–113]. Sirtuin 1 (SIRT1) is a deacetylase involved in normal circadian rhythm modifications, has been linked to increasing longevity, and increases with fasting. Recently NNS's (aspartame and saccharin) were used to suggest the metabolic effects of sugars (not perception of sweetness) resulted in the SIRT1 regulation of a simple sugar preference [114]. It is unknown if NNS consumption during fasting effects such calorie specific pathways as quality of sleep, autophagy, mTOR inhibition, muscle sparing during exercise, or increased efficacy of cancer therapy.

2.4 Effect on cancer

Non-nutritive sweeteners (NNS's) have had a rollercoaster history in being viewed at either increasing or decreasing lifespan, with quality of life being less often measured. An early study by Reuber in 1978, which received tremendous attention in the popular press, appeared to show very high levels of saccahrin causing bladder cancer in rodents [38]. However, earlier and later studies did not support this conclusion and mechanistic data [115] showed different saccharin metabolism in rodents and humans [39, 116, 117]. Yet as a result of the Reuber study, saccharin was listed from 1981 to 2000 as a substance reasonably anticipated to be a human carcinogen in the U.S. National Toxicology Program's Report on Carcinogens [118, 119]. Since 2000 the view of NNS's has increasingly become Generalized Recognized as Safe (GRAS). This continued for maybe 15 years, until recent data showing a failure to reduce obesity has again ramped up questions regarding their utility. However large cohort studies of NNS consumption showed all-cause mortality to increase in a range from 4% [120] - 24% [121]. The correlation with increased risk from cardiovascular (13% [120]) and circulatory disease (52% [121]) was higher.

Recent data suggests that NNS's may actually be beneficial in the treatment of cancer patients [122, 123], in contrast to the earlier attention to carcinogenicity or current concern over obesity in the general public. Cancer cells are well known to be energy hungry, activating molecular pathways of growth to multiply quickly. It has been found that fasting can improve outcomes for cancer patients [123]. The specific food that a cancer patient consumes, or lack thereof, can cause tumor starvation, have cancer-specific toxicity, activate anticancer immune response, or enhance drug-based therapy. Reducing calories have been shown to attack, stress, and kill cancer cells. Low calorie or ketogenic diets increase tumor-infiltrating CD8+ T cells [94, 124] and reduce immune inhibitory ligand expression such as PDL-1138 [125]. If NNS's were used to decrease calories consumed in cancer patients the type and time of remaining calories consumed is still important. Modifying consumption of specific amino acids can be useful when treating cancer patients. For example, both glucose (sugar) and glutamine (protein) are central to cell growth (e.g. TCA cycle, Nucleotide synthesis, Cellular redox balance, Lipid synthesis) [123]. Glucose contributes pyruvate and acetyl-CoA to the TCA cycle while glutamine adds α-ketoglutarate, producing ATP and NADH which is used in oxidative phosphorylation to create even more ATP generation. Both glucose and glutamine are needed for different steps in nucleotide synthesis so lowering consumption of both will synergistically inhibit cancer cells more that inhibition of either alone. Likewise glucose and glutamine work orthogonally to maintain cellular redox potential balance. Glucose is needed for NADPH production via the pentose-phosphate pathway, and glutamine in conjunction with NADPH forms the antioxidant GSH. Lipid synthesis needs both glucose for cytoplasmic acetyl-CoA and glutamine as a carbon source, particularly under hypoxic conditions which are common in tumors. Methionine restriction reduces one-carbon metabolism and nucleotide synthesis, thereby improving cancer inhibition by chemotherapy and radiation. Histidine catabolism reduces cells levels of tetrahydrofolate, which is a cofactor in nucleotide synthesis. The cancer drug Methotrexate inhibits dihydrofolate reductase which generates tetrahydrofolate, therefore histidine supplementation could act synergistically with methotrexate in killing cancer cells [123]. Increasing arginine in mice was found to increase T-cell activation and T-cell mediated antitumor response [126].

All of these example diets with glucose and specific amino acids suggest a cancer patient on a high fat/low carb/low protein diet with NNS's could have better outcomes than if on a normal diet.. While NNS's could increase adherence to such diets it is not currently known if such a diet would be any better than intermittent fasting for cancer patients [95, 98, 105, 127–130], and in fact intermittent fasting has been shown in analysis to have the best adherence of common diets.

NNS's have been shown to increase death, though studies have varied largely in the magnitude of the effect. In 2018 Mulle et al. found NNS's to cause more deaths than natural sugar. The study was done with a 451,743 cohort from across 10 European countries. Participants were fairly healthy and excluded if they had preexisting conditions (cancer, heart disease, stroke, or diabetes at baseline), with a mean (SD) age of 50.8 (9.8) years. The participants were mostly women (71.1%). Participants that consumed 2 or more glasses per day of total soft drinks (with NNS's or sugar beverages, compared to <1 glass per month) died earlier (hazard ratio [HR], 1.17; 95% CI, 1.11–1.22; P < .001). Sugar-sweetened soft drinks only had a HR of 1.08 (95% CI, 1.01–1.16; P = .004), compared to NNS's with a HR of 1.26 (95% CI, 1.16–1.35; P < .001). While NNS's seemed to increase participants risk of deaths from circulatory diseases (HR, 1.52; 95% CI, 1.30–1.78; P < .001), sugar-sweetened soft drinks increased deaths from digestive diseases (HR, 1.59; 95% CI, 1.24–2.05; P < .001) [121].

Some studies have found aspartame to be carcinogenic in large animal studies with rats [131, 132] and mice [131, 133] (many animals per sex and group of exposure, numerous dose levels tested, and with observation extending to death) [134]. In 2012 a prospective epidemiological study showed diet soda with aspartame to increase risk of non-Hodgkin's lymphoma and multiple myeloma in men [135]. Some have theorized that increased aspartame consumption could be linked to an increase in brain tumors [136], but a later study looking at almost half a million people between 50 and 71 years of age found there to be no link between aspartame and either hematopoietic or brain cancer [137]. However, a metaanalysis of 22 studies found aspartame to not cause cancer while looking at low, medium, and high doses in rodents, however it is worth noting that the odds ratio had an extraordinarily large range from 0.115 to 3.500 [138]. While case control studies have found an increased risk of cancer, such as a relative risk (RR) 1.3 for bladder cancer from heavy sweetener consumption, the same study found heavy coffee consumption (50 cups/week) had a RR of 1.4 for bladder cancer [34, 139]. While cancer can result in death, and therefore has large negative effects on Quality of Life Year calculations (QALYs), the data does not suggest NNS's increased cancer risk as much as other diseases, such as circulatory disease and metabolic syndromes.

3. Conclusions

While the continually growing list of NNS's still have many unanswered questions regarding their biological effect in humans, the knowledge we are gaining about each NNS continues to grow as well. Sucralose is now known to become acylated and accumulate in fat tissue. Future studies with sucralose could require long wash out periods, and consumers could expect a delay in biological changes if they removed sucralose from their diet. Aspartame holds a preferential spot among the major NSS's in that it is quickly broken down when consumed so less likely to have some of the deleterious effects by binding sweet receptors outside the oral cavity. Many NNS's alter the gut biome, with sucralose and saccharin seeming particularly deleterious. Unlike aspartame, saccharin is very stable in vivo and binds sweet receptors in the GI tract. Sucralose on the other hand becomes acetylated and accumulates in fat tissue, thereby potentially posing side effects for days long than other NSS's. The altered gut biome reduces satiety, causing consumption of more calories later. Obesity in mice has been alleviated through a fecal transplant which restores the gut biome [140]. This NNS induced dysbiosis also increases digestion of choline, needed for synthesis of VLDL which mobilizes fat from the liver. The choline deficiency and decreased VLDL leads to metabolic issues such as non-alcoholic fatty liver disease (NAFLD) [60].

Future double-blind human studies that would benefit the field would test individual NNS's to determine the causative effect of NNS consumption on:

1. Sleep quality and quantity (when consumed close to sleep)

2. Resting metabolic rate (RMR) during fasting

3. Energy expenditure (EI) during fasting

4. Autophagy during fasting

While the use of NNS's primary goal (reduced obesity) appears discreet, the multiple interacting pathways involved in effecting that change make the cause and effect complex to disentangle (e.g. changing gut biome, leaky gut, NAFLD, increased appetite, decreased RMR).

Conflict of interest

The authors declare no conflict of interest.

Appendices and nomenclature

5-HT	5-hydroxytryptamine, (also) serotonin
Ace-K	Acesulfame-potassium
ADI	Acceptable Daily Intake
ADME	Absorption, Distribution, Metabolism, and Excretion
AUC	Area Under the Curve
CCK	Cholecystokinin
CICO	Calories-In-Calories-Out
CPIR	Cephalic Phase Insulin Response
DMA	Dimethylamine
EC	Enterochromaffin cells
EE	Enteroendocrine cells
FDA	US Food and Drug Administration
GIP	gastric inhibitory peptide, (also) glucose-dependent insulinotropic polypeptide
GERD	Gastroesophageal Reflux Disease
GI	Gastrointestinal
GLP-1	Glucagon-Like Peptide-1
GTT	Glucose Tolerance Test

HbA1C	Glycosylated Hemoglobin
JECFA	Joint Expert Committee on Food Additives
OTUs	Operational Taxonomic Units
OXM	Oxyntomodulin
PAH	Phenylalanine Hydroxylase
PKU	Phenylketonuria
PPP	Pentose Phosphate Pathway
PYY	Peptide Tyrosine Tyrosine
MW	Molecular Weight
NAFLD	Nonalcoholic Fatty Liver Disease
NNS	Non-Nutritional Sweetener
NOAEL	No Observed Adverse Effect Level
QALY	Quality Adjusted Life Year
RR	Relative Risk
SCF	European Union's Scientific Committee for Food
TBW	Total Body Weight
TMA	Trimethylamine
USD	United States of America Dollars
WWTP	Waste Water Treatment Plant

Author details

Sage Arbor
Marian University, Indianapolis, United States

*Address all correspondence to: sagearbor@gmail.com

References

[1] Sylvetsky AC, Jin Y, Clark EJ, Welsh JA, Rother KI, Talegawkar SA. Consumption of Low-Calorie Sweeteners among Children and Adults in the United States. J Acad Nutr Diet. 2017 Mar;117(3):441-448.e2.

[2] Sylvetsky AC, Welsh JA, Brown RJ, Vos MB. Low-calorie sweetener consumption is increasing in the United States123. The American Journal of Clinical Nutrition. 2012 Sep;**96**(3):640-646

[3] Global Artificial Sweetener Market Report 2019: Market Set to Reach $9.7 Billion by 2024 - ResearchAndMarkets.com [Internet]. 2019 [cited 2020 Jun 15]. Available from: https://www.businesswire.com/news/home/20190719005180/en/Global-Artificial-Sweetener-Market-Report-2019-Market

[4] Malek AM, Hunt KJ, DellaValle DM, Greenberg D, St Peter JV, Marriott BP. Reported Consumption of Low-Calorie Sweetener in Foods, Beverages, and Food and Beverage Additions by US Adults: NHANES 2007-2012. Curr Dev Nutr. 2018 Sep;2(9):nzy054.

[5] Kim Y, Keogh JB, Clifton PM. Non-nutritive Sweeteners and Glycaemic Control. Curr Atheroscler Rep. 2019 19;21(12):49.

[6] Benton D, Young HA. Reducing calorie intake may not help you lose body weight. Perspectives on Psychological Science. 2017 Sep 1;**12**(5):703-714

[7] Yoo S. Dynamic energy balance and obesity prevention. J Obes Metab Syndr. 2018 Dec;**27**(4):203-212

[8] Howell S, Kones R. "Calories in, calories out" and macronutrient intake: the hope, hype, and science of calories. Am J Physiol Endocrinol Metab. 2017 01;313(5):E608-12.

[9] Schiffman SS, Rother KI. Sucralose, a synthetic organochlorine sweetener: Overview of biological issues. Journal of Toxicology and Environmental Health. Part B, Critical Reviews. 2013 Sep;**16**(7):399-451

[10] Turner A, Veysey M, Keely S, Scarlett CJ, Lucock M, Beckett EL. Intense Sweeteners, Taste Receptors and the Gut Microbiome: A Metabolic Health Perspective. Int J Environ Res Public Health [Internet]. 2020 Jun [cited 2020 Jul 31];17(11). Available from: https://www.ncbi.nlm.nih.gov/pmc/articles/PMC7312722/

[11] Sugar Substitutes & Non-Nutritive Sweeteners [Internet]. Cleveland Clinic. [cited 2020 Sep 6]. Available from: https://my.clevelandclinic.org/health/articles/15166-sugar-substitutes--non-nutritive-sweeteners

[12] Šedivá A, Panovská Z, Pokorný J. Sensory profiles of sweeteners in aqueous solutions. Czech Journal of Food Sciences. 2006;**24**:283-287

[13] Tan VWK, Wee MSM, Tomic O, Forde CG. Temporal sweetness and side tastes profiles of 16 sweeteners using temporal check-all-that-apply (TCATA). Food Research International. 2019 Jul 1;**121**:39-47

[14] Harrington EO, Vang A, Braza J, Shil A, Chichger H. Activation of the sweet taste receptor, T1R3, by the artificial sweetener sucralose regulates the pulmonary endothelium. American Journal of Physiology. Lung Cellular and Molecular Physiology. 2018 Jan 1;**314**(1):L165-L176

[15] Mahalapbutr P, Darai N, Panman W, Opasmahakul A, Kungwan N, Hannongbua S, et al. Atomistic mechanisms underlying the activation of the G protein-coupled sweet receptor heterodimer by sugar alcohol

recognition. Sci Rep [Internet]. 2019 Jul 15 [cited 2020 Aug 3];9. Available from: https://www.ncbi.nlm.nih.gov/pmc/articles/PMC6629994/

[16] Nutrition C for FS and A. Additional Information about High-Intensity Sweeteners Permitted for Use in Food in the United States. FDA [Internet]. 2020 Feb 20 [cited 2020 Aug 3]; Available from: https://www.fda.gov/food/food-additives-petitions/additional-information-about-high-intensity-sweeteners-permitted-use-food-united-states

[17] Wheeler A, Boileau AC, Winkler PC, Compton JC, Prakash I, Jiang X, et al. Pharmacokinetics of rebaudioside a and stevioside after single oral doses in healthy men. Food and Chemical Toxicology. 2008 Jul;**46**(Suppl 7):S54-S60

[18] Geuns JMC, Buyse J, Vankeirsbilck A, Temme EHM, Compernolle F, Toppet S. Identification of steviol glucuronide in human urine. Journal of Agricultural and Food Chemistry. 2006 Apr 5;**54**(7): 2794-2798

[19] Sweeteners, High-Intensity - Chemical Economics Handbook (CEH) | IHS Markit [Internet]. [cited 2020 Sep 2]. Available from: https://ihsmarkit.com/products/high-intensity-sweeteners-chemical-economics-handbook.html

[20] Petersson S. Where Do Sugar and Sweeteners Stand Today [Internet]. Market Research Blog. 2017 [cited 2020 Sep 2]. Available from: https://blog.euromonitor.com/where-do-sugar-sweeteners-stand-today/

[21] Luo J, Zhang Q, Cao M, Wu L, Cao J, Fang F, et al. Ecotoxicity and environmental fates of newly recognized contaminants-artificial sweeteners: A review. Sci Total Environ. 2019 Feb 25;**653**:1149-1160

[22] Praveena SM, Cheema MS, Guo H-R. Non-nutritive artificial sweeteners as an emerging contaminant in environment: A global review and risks perspectives. Ecotoxicology and Environmental Safety. 2019 Apr 15;**170**:699-707

[23] Tran NH, Hu J, Li J, Ong SL. Suitability of artificial sweeteners as indicators of raw wastewater contamination in surface water and groundwater. Water Research. 2014 Jan 1;**48**:443-456

[24] Lubick N. Artificial sweetener persists in the environment. Environmental Science & Technology. 2008 May 1;**42**(9):3125-3125

[25] Brown RJ, De Banate MA, Rother KI. Artificial sweeteners: A systematic review of metabolic effects in youth. International Journal of Pediatric Obesity. 2010 Aug;**5**(4):305-312

[26] Findikli Z, Turkoglu S. Determination of the effects of some artificial sweeteners on human peripheral lymphocytes using the comet assay. JTEHS. 2014 Oct 31;**6**(8):147-153

[27] Belton K, Schaefer E. Guiney PD. Integr Environ Assess Manag: A Review of the Environmental Fate and Effects of Acesulfame-Potassium; 2020 Feb 17

[28] JJ M. Absorption and Metabolism of Sugar Substitutes (Artificial Sweeteners) | Aspartame, Sucralose, Etc. [Internet]. 2018 [cited 2020 Aug 1]. Available from: https://www.youtube.com/watch?v=CCBcsNaep-g

[29] Marie S. Piggott JR. Springer Science & Business Media: Handbook of Sweeteners; 2013. 316 p

[30] Bernstein LE, Rohr F, Helm JR, editors. Nutrition Management of Inherited Metabolic Diseases: Lessons from Metabolic University [Internet]. Springer International Publishing; 2015 [cited 2020 Aug 1]. Available from: http://www.springer.com/gp/book/9783319146201

[31] Brosco JP, Sanders LM, Seider MI, Dunn AC. Adverse medical outcomes of early newborn screening programs for phenylketonuria. Pediatrics. 2008 Jul 1;**122**(1):192-197

[32] Trefz KF, Muntau AC, Kohlscheen KM, Altevers J, Jacob C, Braun S, et al. Clinical burden of illness in patients with phenylketonuria (PKU) and associated comorbidities - a retrospective study of German health insurance claims data. Orphanet Journal of Rare Diseases. 2019 Jul 22;**14**(1):181

[33] Burton BK, Jones KB, Cederbaum S, Rohr F, Waisbren S, Irwin DE, et al. Prevalence of comorbid conditions among adult patients diagnosed with phenylketonuria. Molecular Genetics and Metabolism. 2018 Nov 1;**125**(3):228-234

[34] Weihrauch MR, Diehl V. Artificial sweeteners--do they bear a carcinogenic risk? Annals of Oncology. 2004 Oct;**15**(10):1460-1465

[35] Stegink LD, Brummel MC, McMartin K, Martin-Amat G, Filer LJ, Baker GL, et al. Blood methanol concentrations in normal adult subjects administered abuse doses of aspartame. Journal of Toxicology and Environmental Health. 1981 Feb;**7**(2):281-290

[36] Butchko HH, Stargel WW, Comer CP, Mayhew DA, Benninger C, Blackburn GL, et al. Aspartame: Review of safety. Regulatory Toxicology and Pharmacology. 2002 Apr;**35**(2 Pt 2): S1-S93

[37] Sathyapalan T, Thatcher NJ, Hammersley R, Rigby AS, Courts FL, Pechlivanis A, et al. Aspartame sensitivity? A double blind randomised crossover study. PLoS One. 2015;**10**(3): e0116212

[38] Reuber MD. Carcinogenicity of saccharin. Environmental Health Perspectives. 1978 Aug;**25**:173-200

[39] Chappel CI. A review and biological risk assessment of sodium saccharin. Regulatory Toxicology and Pharmacology. 1992 Jun;**15**(3):253-270

[40] Arnold DL, Krewski D, Munro IC. Saccharin: A toxicological and historical perspective. Toxicology. 1983 Aug;**27**(3-4):179-256

[41] Renwick AG. The intake of intense sweeteners - an update review. Food Additives and Contaminants. 2006 Apr;**23**(4):327-338

[42] Renwick AG. The use of a sweetener substitution method to predict dietary exposures for the intense sweetener rebaudioside a. Food and Chemical Toxicology. 2008 Jul;**46**(Suppl 7):S61-S69

[43] Organization WH, Nations F and AO of the U, Joint FAO/WHO Expert Committee on Food Additives. Meeting (80th: 2015 R. Evaluation of certain food additives and contaminants: eightieth report of the Joint FAO/WHO Expert Committee on Food Additives [Internet]. World Health Organization; 2016 [cited 2020 Aug 7]. Available from: https://apps.who.int/iris/handle/10665/204410

[44] Horne J, Lawless HT, Speirs W, Sposato D. Bitter taste of saccharin and acesulfame-K. Chemical Senses. 2002 Jan 1;**27**(1):31-38

[45] Azad MB, Abou-Setta AM, Chauhan BF, Rabbani R, Lys J, Copstein L, et al. Nonnutritive sweeteners and cardiometabolic health: A systematic review and meta-analysis of randomized controlled trials and prospective cohort studies. CMAJ. 2017 Jul 17;**189**(28):E929-E939

[46] Kuk JL, Brown RE. Aspartame intake is associated with greater glucose intolerance in individuals with obesity. Applied Physiology, Nutrition, and Metabolism. 2016 Jul;**41**(7):795-798

[47] Swithers SE. Artificial sweeteners produce the counterintuitive effect

of inducing metabolic derangements. Trends in Endocrinology and Metabolism. 2013 Sep;**24**(9):431-441

[48] Symonds ME, Sebert SP, Hyatt MA, Budge H. Nutritional programming of the metabolic syndrome. Nature Reviews. Endocrinology. 2009 Nov;**5**(11):604-610

[49] Chattopadhyay S, Raychaudhuri U, Chakraborty R. Artificial sweeteners – A review. Journal of Food Science and Technology. 2014 Apr;**51**(4):611-621

[50] Klug C, von Rymon Lipinski G-W. Acesulfame K [Internet]. ResearchGate. [cited 2020 Aug 7]. Available from: https://www.researchgate.net/publication/277693817_Acesulfame_K

[51] Food Additives Permitted for Direct Addition to Food for Human Consumption; Acesulfame Potassium [Internet]. Federal Register. 2003 [cited 2020 Aug 7]. Available from: https://www.federalregister.gov/documents/2003/12/31/03-32101/food-additives-permitted-for-direct-addition-to-food-for-human-consumption-acesulfame-potassium

[52] 706. Introduction (WHO Food Additives Series 28) [Internet]. [cited 2020 Aug 7]. Available from: http://www.inchem.org/documents/jecfa/jecmono/v28je01.htm

[53] Sharma VK, Oturan M, Kim H. Oxidation of artificial sweetener sucralose by advanced oxidation processes: A review. Environmental Science and Pollution Research. 2014 Jul 1;**21**(14):8525-8533

[54] Berry C, Brusick D, Cohen SM, Hardisty JF, Grotz VL, Williams GM. Sucralose non-carcinogenicity: A review of the scientific and regulatory rationale. Nutrition and Cancer. 2016 Nov 16;**68**(8):1247-1261

[55] John BA, Wood SG, Hawkins DR. The pharmacokinetics and metabolism of sucralose in the mouse. Food and Chemical Toxicology. 2000;**38**(Suppl 2): S107-S110

[56] Roberts A, Renwick AG, Sims J, Snodin DJ. Sucralose metabolism and pharmacokinetics in man. Food and Chemical Toxicology. 2000;**38**(Suppl 2): S31-S41

[57] Grice HC, Goldsmith LA. Sucralose--an overview of the toxicity data. Food and Chemical Toxicology. 2000;**38**(Suppl 2):S1-S6

[58] Rother KI, Conway EM, Sylvetsky AC. How non-nutritive sweeteners influence hormones and health. Trends in Endocrinology & Metabolism. 2018 Jul 1;**29**(7):455-467

[59] Ko J-A, Ryu YB, Kwon H-J, Jeong HJ, Park S-J, Kim CY, et al. Characterization of a novel steviol-producing β-glucosidase from Penicillium decumbens and optimal production of the steviol. Applied Microbiology and Biotechnology. 2013 Sep;**97**(18):8151-8161

[60] Emamat H, Ghalandari H, Tangestani H, Abdollahi A, Hekmatdoost A. Artificial sweeteners are related to non-alcoholic fatty liver disease: Microbiota dysbiosis as a novel potential mechanism. EXCLI Journal. 2020;**19**:620-626

[61] Suez J, Korem T, Zeevi D, Zilberman-Schapira G, Thaiss CA, Maza O, et al. Artificial sweeteners induce glucose intolerance by altering the gut microbiota. Nature [Internet]. 2014 Sep 17 [cited 2014 Sep 25];advance online publication. Available from: http://www.nature.com/nature/journal/vaop/ncurrent/full/nature13793.html

[62] Ruiz-Ojeda FJ, Plaza-Díaz J, Sáez-Lara MJ, Gil A. Effects of Sweeteners on the Gut Microbiota: A Review of Experimental Studies and Clinical Trials. Adv Nutr. 2019 Jan 1;10(suppl_1):S31-48.

[63] Uebanso T, Ohnishi A, Kitayama R, Yoshimoto A, Nakahashi M, Shimohata T, et al. Effects of Low-Dose Non-Caloric Sweetener Consumption on Gut Microbiota in Mice. Nutrients [Internet]. 2017 Jun 1 [cited 2020 Jul 16];9(6). Available from: https://www.ncbi.nlm.nih.gov/pmc/articles/PMC5490539/

[64] Lobach AR, Roberts A, Rowland IR. Assessing the in vivo data on low/no-calorie sweeteners and the gut microbiota. Food and Chemical Toxicology. 2019 Feb;**124**:385-399

[65] Mandrioli D, Kearns CE, Bero LA. Relationship between Research Outcomes and Risk of Bias, Study Sponsorship, and Author Financial Conflicts of Interest in Reviews of the Effects of Artificially Sweetened Beverages on Weight Outcomes: A Systematic Review of Reviews. PLoS One [Internet]. 2016 Sep 8 [cited 2019 May 10];11(9). Available from: https://www.ncbi.nlm.nih.gov/pmc/articles/PMC5015869/

[66] Plaza-Diaz J, Pastor-Villaescusa B, Rueda-Robles A, Abadia-Molina F, Ruiz-Ojeda FJ. Plausible Biological Interactions of Low- and Non-Calorie Sweeteners with the Intestinal Microbiota: An Update of Recent Studies. Nutrients [Internet]. 2020 Apr 21 [cited 2020 Jun 5];12(4). Available from: https://www.ncbi.nlm.nih.gov/pmc/articles/PMC7231174/

[67] Gultekin F, Oner ME, Savas HB, Dogan B. Food additives and microbiota. North Clin Istanb. 2019 Jul 17;**7**(2): 192-200

[68] Bornemann V, Werness SC, Buslinger L, Schiffman SS. Intestinal metabolism and bioaccumulation of sucralose In adipose tissue In the rat. Journal of Toxicology and Environmental Health, Part A. 2018 Sep 17;**81**(18):913-923

[69] Ojeda P, Bobe A, Dolan K, Leone V, Martinez K. Nutritional modulation of gut microbiota - the impact on metabolic disease pathophysiology. The Journal of Nutritional Biochemistry. 2016 Feb;**28**:191-200

[70] Corbin KD, Zeisel SH. The Nutrigenetics and Nutrigenomics of the Dietary Requirement for Choline. In: Bouchard C, Ordovas JM, editors. Progress in Molecular Biology and Translational Science [Internet]. Academic Press; 2012 [cited 2018 Mar 12]. p. 159-77. (Recent Advances in Nutrigenetics and Nutrigenomics; vol. 108). Available from: http://www.sciencedirect.com/science/article/pii/B9780123983978000071

[71] Corbin KD, Zeisel SH. Choline metabolism provides novel insights into non-alcoholic fatty liver disease and its progression. Current Opinion in Gastroenterology. 2012 Mar;**28**(2):159-165

[72] Fowler SP, Williams K, Resendez RG, Hunt KJ, Hazuda HP, Stern MP. Fueling the obesity epidemic? Artificially sweetened beverage use and long-term weight gain. Obesity (Silver Spring). 2008 Aug;**16**(8):1894-1900

[73] Veldhuizen MG, Babbs RK, Patel B, Fobbs W, Kroemer NB, Garcia E, et al. Integration of sweet taste and metabolism determines carbohydrate reward. Curr Biol. 2017 Aug 21;27(16):2476-2485.e6.

[74] Martin AM, Sun EW, Keating DJ. Mechanisms controlling hormone secretion in human gut and its relevance to metabolism. The Journal of Endocrinology. 2019 Nov 18;**244**(1):R1-R15

[75] Martin AM, Lumsden AL, Young RL, Jessup CF, Spencer NJ, Keating DJ. Regional differences in nutrient-induced secretion of gut serotonin. Physiol Rep. 2017 Mar;5(6).

[76] Zelkas L, Raghupathi R, Lumsden AL, Martin AM, Sun E,

Spencer NJ, et al. Serotonin-secreting enteroendocrine cells respond via diverse mechanisms to acute and chronic changes in glucose availability. Nutrition & Metabolism. 2015 Dec 15;**12**(1):55

[77] Kidd M, Modlin IM, Gustafsson BI, Drozdov I, Hauso O, Pfragner R. Luminal regulation of normal and neoplastic human EC cell serotonin release is mediated by bile salts, amines, tastants, and olfactants. American Journal of Physiology - Gastrointestinal and Liver Physiology. 2008 Aug 1;**295**(2):G260-G272

[78] Yano JM, Yu K, Donaldson GP, Shastri GG, Ann P, Ma L, et al. Indigenous bacteria from the gut microbiota regulate host serotonin biosynthesis. Cell. 2015 Apr 9;**161**(2):264-276

[79] Crane JD, Palanivel R, Mottillo EP, Bujak AL, Wang H, Ford RJ, et al. Inhibiting peripheral serotonin synthesis reduces obesity and metabolic dysfunction by promoting brown adipose tissue thermogenesis. Nature Medicine. 2015 Feb;**21**(2):166-172

[80] Young RL, Lumsden AL, Martin AM, Schober G, Pezos N, Thazhath SS, et al. Augmented capacity for peripheral serotonin release in human obesity. International Journal of Obesity. 2018;**42**(11):1880-1889

[81] Young J, Conway EM, Rother KI, Sylvetsky AC. Low-calorie sweetener use, weight, and metabolic health among children: A mini-review. Pediatric Obesity. 2019;**14**(8):e12521

[82] Teff KL, Mattes RD, Engelman K. Cephalic phase insulin release in normal weight males: Verification and reliability. The American Journal of Physiology. 1991 Oct;**261**(4 Pt 1): E430-E436

[83] Yamazaki M, Sakaguchi T. Effects of D-glucose anomers on sweetness taste and insulin release in man. Brain Research Bulletin. 1986 Aug 1;**17**(2):271-274

[84] Dhillon J, Lee JY, Mattes RD. The cephalic phase insulin response to nutritive and low-calorie sweeteners in solid and beverage form. Physiology & Behavior. 2017 Nov 1;**181**:100-109

[85] Smeets PA, de Graaf C, Stafleu A, van Osch MJ, van der Grond J. Functional magnetic resonance imaging of human hypothalamic responses to sweet taste and calories. The American Journal of Clinical Nutrition. 2005 Nov 1;**82**(5):1011-1016

[86] Härtel B, Graubaum H. Schneider B. The Influence of Sweetener Solutions on the Secretion of Insulin and the Blood Glucose Level. In 2012

[87] Glendinning JI, Frim YG, Hochman A, Lubitz GS, Basile AJ, Sclafani A. Glucose elicits cephalic-phase insulin release in mice by activating KATP channels in taste cells. American Journal of Physiology-Regulatory, Integrative and Comparative Physiology. 2017 Jan 27;**312**(4):R597-R610

[88] Yee KK, Sukumaran SK, Kotha R, Gilbertson TA, Margolskee RF. Glucose transporters and ATP-gated K+ (KATP) metabolic sensors are present in type 1 taste receptor 3 (T1r3)-expressing taste cells. PNAS. 2011 Mar 29;**108**(13):5431-5436

[89] Jaspers RT, Zillikens MC, Friesema ECH. Delli Paoli G, Bloch W, Uitterlinden AG, et al. exercise, fasting, and mimetics: Toward beneficial combinations? The FASEB Journal. 2017;**31**(1):14-28

[90] Lee S, Dong HH. FoxO integration of insulin signaling with glucose and lipid metabolism. The Journal of Endocrinology. 2017 May 1;**233**(2):R67-R79

[91] Kim I, Lemasters JJ. Mitochondrial degradation by autophagy (mitophagy)

in GFP-LC3 transgenic hepatocytes during nutrient deprivation. American Journal of Physiology. Cell Physiology. 2011 Feb;**300**(2):C308-C317

[92] Alirezaei M, Kemball CC, Flynn CT, Wood MR, Whitton JL, Kiosses WB. Short-term fasting induces profound neuronal autophagy. Autophagy. 2010 Aug 16;**6**(6):702-710

[93] O'Rourke EJ, Kuballa P, Xavier R, Ruvkun G. ω-6 polyunsaturated fatty acids extend life span through the activation of autophagy. Genes & Development. 2013 Feb 15;**27**(4):429-440

[94] Pietrocola F, Pol J, Vacchelli E, Rao S, Enot DP, Baracco EE, et al. Caloric restriction Mimetics enhance anticancer immunosurveillance. Cancer Cell. 2016 Jul 11;**30**(1):147-160

[95] Hanjani NA, Vafa M. Protein Restriction, Epigenetic Diet. Intermittent Fasting as New Approaches for Preventing Age-associated Diseases. Int J Prev Med. 2018;**9**:58

[96] Hillson O, Gonzalez S, Rallis C. Prospects of pharmacological interventions to organismal aging. Biomolecular Concepts. 2018 Dec 31;**9**(1):200-215

[97] Kincaid B, Bossy-Wetzel E. Forever young: SIRT3 a shield against mitochondrial meltdown, aging, and neurodegeneration. Front Aging Neurosci [Internet]. 2013 Sep 6 [cited 2015 Jan 21];5. Available from: http://www.ncbi.nlm.nih.gov/pmc/articles/PMC3764375/

[98] Francesco AD, Germanio CD, Bernier M, Cabo R de. A time to fast. Science 2018 Nov 16;362(6416):770-775.

[99] Arbor S. Where and How in the mTOR Pathway Inhibitors Fight Aging: Rapamycin, Resveratrol, and Metformin. Resveratrol - Adding Life to Years, Not Adding Years to Life [Internet]. 2018 Nov 5 [cited 2019 Feb 6]; Available from: https://www.intechopen.com/books/resveratrol-adding-life-to-years-not-adding-years-to-life/where-and-how-in-the-mtor-pathway-inhibitors-fight-aging-rapamycin-resveratrol-and-metformin

[100] Arbor SC, LaFontaine M, Cumbay M. Amyloid-beta Alzheimer targets — Protein processing, lipid rafts, and amyloid-beta pores. The Yale Journal of Biology and Medicine. 2016 Mar 24;**89**(1):5-21

[101] Xu K, Morgan KT, Todd Gehris A, Elston TC, Gomez SM. A Whole-Body Model for Glycogen Regulation Reveals a Critical Role for Substrate Cycling in Maintaining Blood Glucose Homeostasis. PLoS Comput Biol [Internet]. 2011 Dec 1 [cited 2018 Oct 8];7(12). Available from: https://www.ncbi.nlm.nih.gov/pmc/articles/PMC3233304/

[102] Longo VD, Panda S. Fasting, circadian rhythms, and time restricted feeding in healthy lifespan. Cell Metabolism. 2016 Jun 14;**23**(6):1048-1059

[103] Mattson MP, Moehl K, Ghena N, Schmaedick M, Cheng A. Intermittent metabolic switching, neuroplasticity and brain health. Nature Reviews. Neuroscience. 2018 Feb;**19**(2):63-80

[104] Heilbronn LK, Civitarese AE, Bogacka I, Smith SR, Hulver M, Ravussin E. Glucose tolerance and skeletal muscle gene expression in response to alternate day fasting. Obesity Research. 2005 Mar;**13**(3):574-581

[105] Alhamdan BA, Garcia-Alvarez A, Alzahrnai AH, Karanxha J, Stretchberry DR, Contrera KJ, et al. Alternate-day versus daily energy restriction diets: Which is more effective for weight loss? A systematic review and meta-analysis. Obesity Science and Practice. 2016 Sep;**2**(3):293-302

[106] Ahmet I, Tae H-J, de Cabo R, Lakatta EG, Talan MI. Effects of calorie restriction on Cardioprotection and cardiovascular health. Journal of Molecular and Cellular Cardiology. 2011 Aug;**51**(2):263-271

[107] Harris L, Hamilton S, Azevedo LB, Olajide J, De Brún C, Waller G, et al. Intermittent fasting interventions for treatment of overweight and obesity in adults: A systematic review and meta-analysis. JBI Database of Systematic Reviews and Implementation Reports. 2018 Feb;**16**(2):507-547

[108] Zhang L, Cordeiro LS, Liu J, Ma Y. The Association between Breakfast Skipping and Body Weight, Nutrient Intake, and Metabolic Measures among Participants with Metabolic Syndrome. Nutrients [Internet]. 2017 Apr 14;9(4). Available from: http://www.ncbi.nlm.nih.gov/pmc/articles/PMC5409723/

[109] Furmli S, Elmasry R, Ramos M, Fung J. Therapeutic use of intermittent fasting for people with type 2 diabetes as an alternative to insulin. BMJ Case Reports. 2018 Oct 9;2018:bcr-2017-221854.

[110] Schwingshackl L, Schlesinger S, Devleesschauwer B, Hoffmann G, Bechthold A, Schwedhelm C, et al. Generatingtheevidenceforriskreduction: A contribution to the future of food-based dietary guidelines. The Proceedings of the Nutrition Society. 2018;**77**(4):432-444

[111] Long MW, Gortmaker SL, Ward ZJ, Resch SC, Moodie ML, Sacks G, et al. Cost effectiveness of a sugar-sweetened beverage excise tax in the U.S. American Journal of Preventive Medicine. 2015 Jul;**49**(1):112-123

[112] Wilde P, Huang Y, Sy S, Abrahams-Gessel S, Jardim TV, Paarlberg R, et al. Cost-effectiveness of a US National Sugar-Sweetened Beverage tax with a multistakeholder approach: Who pays and who benefits. American Journal of Public Health. 2019;**109**(2):276-284

[113] Lee Y, Mozaffarian D, Liu J, Sy S, Abrahams-Gessel S, Wilde P, et al. Health Impact and Cost-effectiveness of Volume, Tiered, and Sugar Content Sugar-sweetened Beverage Tax Policies in the US: A Micro-simulation Study (OR28-04-19). Curr Dev Nutr [Internet]. 2019 Jun 1 [cited 2020 Sep 3];3(Supplement_1). Available from: https://academic.oup.com/cdn/article/3/Supplement_1/nzz042.OR28-04-19/5518172

[114] Matsui S, Sasaki T, Kohno D, Yaku K, Inutsuka A, Yokota-Hashimoto H, et al. Neuronal SIRT1 regulates macronutrient-based diet selection through FGF21 and oxytocin signalling in mice. Nature Communications. 2018 Nov 2;**9**(1):4604

[115] Cohen SM, Cano M, Earl RA, Carson SD, Garland EM. A proposed role for silicates and protein in the proliferative effects of saccharin on the male rat urothelium. Carcinogenesis. 1991 Sep;**12**(9):1551-1555

[116] Whysner J, Williams GM. Saccharin mechanistic data and risk assessment: Urine composition, enhanced cell proliferation, and tumor promotion. Pharmacology & Therapeutics. 1996;**71**(1-2):225-252

[117] Elcock M, Morgan RW. Update on artificial sweeteners and bladder cancer. Regulatory Toxicology and Pharmacology. 1993 Feb;**17**(1):35-43

[118] NTP (National Toxicology Program). Report on Carcinogens, Fourteenth Edition [Internet]. 2016. Available from: http://ntp.niehs.nih.gov/go/roc14

[119] Serra-Majem L, Raposo A, Aranceta-Bartrina J, Varela-Moreiras G, Logue C, Laviada H, et al. Ibero–American Consensus on Low- and No-Calorie Sweeteners: Safety, Nutritional Aspects and Benefits

in Food and Beverages. Nutrients [Internet]. 2018 Jun 25 [cited 2020 Jul 17];10(7). Available from: https://www.ncbi.nlm.nih.gov/pmc/articles/PMC6073242/

[120] Malik VS, Li Y, Pan A, De Koning L, Schernhammer E, Willett WC, et al. Long-Term Consumption of Sugar-Sweetened and Artificially Sweetened Beverages and Risk of Mortality in US Adults. Circulation. 2019 30;139(18): 2113-25.

[121] Mullee A, Romaguera D, Pearson-Stuttard J, Viallon V, Stepien M, Freisling H, et al. Association between soft drink consumption and mortality in 10 European countries. JAMA Internal Medicine. 2019 Nov 1;**179**(11):1479-1490

[122] O'Flanagan CH, Smith LA, McDonell SB, Hursting SD. When less may be more: calorie restriction and response to cancer therapy. BMC Med [Internet]. 2017 May 24 [cited 2018 Aug 23];15. Available from: https://www.ncbi.nlm.nih.gov/pmc/articles/PMC5442682/

[123] Kanarek N, Petrova B, Sabatini DM. Dietary modifications for enhanced cancer therapy. Nature. 2020;**579**(7800):507-517

[124] Di Biase S, Lee C, Brandhorst S, Manes B, Buono R, Cheng C-W, et al. Fasting mimicking diet reduces HO-1 to promote T cell-mediated tumor cytotoxicity. Cancer Cell. 2016 Jul 11;**30**(1):136-146

[125] Lussier DM, Woolf EC, Johnson JL, Brooks KS, Blattman JN, Scheck AC. Enhanced immunity in a mouse model of malignant glioma is mediated by a therapeutic ketogenic diet. BMC Cancer [Internet]. 2016 May 13 [cited 2020 Jul 17];16. Available from: https://www.ncbi.nlm.nih.gov/pmc/articles/PMC4866042/

[126] Geiger R, Rieckmann JC, Wolf T, Basso C, Feng Y, Fuhrer T, et al. L-Arginine Modulates T Cell Metabolism and Enhances Survival and Anti-tumor Activity. Cell. 2016 Oct 20;167(3):829-842.e13.

[127] Koliaki C, Spinos T, Spinou M, Brinia M-E, Mitsopoulou D, Katsilambros N, et al. Defining the optimal dietary approach for safe, effective and sustainable weight loss in overweight and obese adults. Healthcare. 2018 Jun 28;**6**(3):73

[128] Cioffi I, Evangelista A, Ponzo V, Ciccone G, Soldati L, Santarpia L, et al. Intermittent versus continuous energy restriction on weight loss and cardiometabolic outcomes: A systematic review and meta-analysis of randomized controlled trials. Journal of Translational Medicine. 2018 Dec 24;**16**(1):371

[129] Chowdhury EA, Richardson JD, Tsintzas K, Thompson D, Betts JA. Effect of extended morning fasting upon ad libitum lunch intake and associated metabolic and hormonal responses in obese adults. International Journal of Obesity. 2016 Feb;**40**(2):305-311

[130] Mallik R, Chowdhury TA. Metformin in cancer. Diabetes Research and Clinical Practice [Internet]. [cited 2018 May 31]; Available from: https://www.sciencedirect.com/science/article/pii/S0168822717314109

[131] Soffritti M, Belpoggi F, Esposti DD, Lambertini L, Tibaldi E, Rigano A. First experimental demonstration of the multipotential carcinogenic effects of aspartame administered in the feed to Sprague-Dawley rats. Environmental Health Perspectives. 2006 Mar;**114**(3):379-385

[132] Soffritti M, Belpoggi F, Tibaldi E, Esposti DD, Lauriola M. Life-span exposure to low doses of aspartame beginning during prenatal life increases cancer effects in rats.

Environmental Health Perspectives. 2007 Sep;**115**(9):1293-1297

[133] Soffritti M, Belpoggi F, Manservigi M, Tibaldi E, Lauriola M, Falcioni L, et al. Aspartame administered in feed, beginning prenatally through life span, induces cancers of the liver and lung in male Swiss mice. American Journal of Industrial Medicine. 2010 Dec;**53**(12):1197-1206

[134] Soffritti M, Belpoggi F, Minardi F, Bua L, Maltoni C. Mega-experiments to identify and assess diffuse carcinogenic risks. Annals of the New York Academy of Sciences. 1999;**895**:34-55

[135] Schernhammer ES, Bertrand KA, Birmann BM, Sampson L, Willett WC, Feskanich D. Consumption of artificial sweetener- and sugar-containing soda and risk of lymphoma and leukemia in men and women1234. The American Journal of Clinical Nutrition. 2012 Dec;**96**(6):1419-1428

[136] Olney JW, Farber NB, Spitznagel E, Robins LN. Increasing brain tumor rates: Is there a link to aspartame? Journal of Neuropathology and Experimental Neurology. 1996 Nov;**55**(11):1115-1123

[137] Lim U, Subar AF, Mouw T, Hartge P, Morton LM, Stolzenberg-Solomon R, et al. Consumption of aspartame-containing beverages and incidence of hematopoietic and brain malignancies. Cancer Epidemiology, Biomarkers & Prevention. 2006 Sep;**15**(9):1654-1659

[138] Mallikarjun S, Sieburth RM. Aspartame and risk of cancer: A meta-analytic review. Archives of Environmental & Occupational Health. 2015 May 4;**70**(3):133-141

[139] Sturgeon SR, Hartge P, Silverman DT, Kantor AF, Linehan WM, Lynch C, et al. Associations between bladder cancer risk factors and tumor stage and grade at diagnosis. Epidemiology. 1994 Mar;**5**(2):218-225

[140] Liou AP, Paziuk M, Luevano J-M, Machineni S, Turnbaugh PJ, Kaplan LM. Conserved shifts in the gut microbiota due to gastric bypass reduce host weight and adiposity. Sci Transl Med. 2013 Mar 27;5(178):178ra41.

Chapter 5

Hyperglycemia- and Hyperlipidemia-Induced Inflammation and Oxidative Stress through Human T Lymphocytes and Human Aortic Endothelial Cells (HAEC)

Frankie B. Stentz

Abstract

Approximately 65% of patients with T2DM die as a result of cardiovascular disease with hyperglycemia and hyperlipidemia being important risk factors for cardiovascular diseases. Both T2DM and atherosclerosis are considered to be inflammatory processes Human T-lymphocytes (T-cells) and aortic endothelial cells (HAEC) have been shown to be components of plaque formation in atherosclerosis. T cells and HAEC are unique in that in their naive state they have no insulin receptors responsive to insulin but become activated in vitro hyperglycemia and in vivo hyperglycemic conditions such as diabetic ketoacidosis and non-ketotic hyperglycemic conditions. Our studies show that T-cells and HAEC in the presence of high concentrations of glucose /and or the saturated fatty acid (SFA) palmitic acid become activated and express insulin receptors, reactive oxygen species (ROS), cytokine elevation, and lipid peroxidation in a time and concentration-dependent manner. Whereas, the unsaturated fatty acid α-linoleic, was not able to activate these cells and had a salutary effect on the activation by glucose and palmitic acid. We have demonstrated that unsaturated fatty acids (UFA) may provide a protective mechanism against the prooxidant effects of hyperglycemia and high SFA such as palmitic acid. Therefore, diet alternations may be beneficial for decreasing hyperglycemia and cardiovascular risks. Studies have shown that lifestyle changes of diet and exercise can reduce the risk of developing diabetes by 58%. Hyperglycemia and hyperlipidemia are important risk factors of developing diabetes and cardiovascular disease. Therefore, we studied the effects of a High Protein diet versus a High Carbohydrate diet in obese non-diabetic, prediabetic and diabetic subjects for effects on weight loss, blood sugar, lipid levels, inflammation, and oxidative stress.

Keywords: blood glucose, free fatty acids, insulin sensitivity, inflammation, cardiovascular risk factors, T lymphocytes, human aortic endothelial cells (HAEC), high protein diet (HP), high carbohydrate diet (HC)

1. Introduction

Greater than 65% of patients with Type 2 Diabetes Mellitus (T2DM) die as a result of cardiovascular disease with hyperglycemia and hyperlipidemia being important risk factors for cardiovascular diseases [1]. Studies have shown that glucose control results in reduction in risk of microvascular complications in diabetes mellitus [2]. The relationship between hyperglycemia and macrovascular complications, however, is not as evident even though subjects with T2DM are two to four times more prone to develop cardiovascular pathology than nondiabetic subjects [3, 4]. Hyperglycemia is a crucial factor contributing to vascular impairment in diabetes mellitus, obesity, and metabolic syndrome [2, 5–7]. Evidence indicates that in hyperglycemic conditions a major contributor to development of large vessel pathology is the endothelial dysfunction [8–10]. Studies have shown that hyperglycemia impairs insulin induced vasodilatory action by decreasing endothelial cells ability to activate nitric oxide synthase-nitric oxide pathway [11]. In hyperglycemic crisis of Diabetic Ketoacidosis (DKA) or hyperglycemic nonketotic state, where both hyperglycemia and high fatty acids are elevated, levels of proinflammatory cytokines and oxidative stress are stimulated [12].

Both T2DM and atherosclerosis are considered to be inflammatory processes [13]. Human T-lymphocytes (T-cells) have been shown to be components of plaque formation along with endothelial cells in atherosclerosis [13]. Human T-lymphocytes have unique properties in that in their naïve state they are insulin unresponsive but upon exposure to high glucose levels they become activated and develop insulin receptors (INR) with emergence of insulin degrading enzyme and insulin responsive glucose uptake [14–19]. Our studies have shown that reactive oxygen species (ROS) along with proinflammatory cytokines such as: Tumor Necrosis Factor α (TNF-α), Interleukin-6 (IL-6), Interleukin-1β (IL-1β) and Interleukin-8 (IL-8); cardiovascular risk markers such as: PAI-1, CRP and Free Fatty Acids (FFA); and counterregulatory hormones such as: IGF-1 and cortisol were all elevated two to three fold above normal with hyperglycemia and returned to normal levels after resolution of hyperglycemia with treatment with insulin and hydration [12]. Our studies have also shown in vitro effects of hyperglycemia (15 and 30 mM) on activation of T-lymphocytes by emergence of IGF-1, INR and Vitamin D receptors and increased levels of ROS and lipid peroxidation [15–18, 20].

Human aortic endothelial cells (HAEC) are also unique in that in their native unstimulated state of glucose of 5 mM they are insulin non-responsive, with GLUT1 as the major glucose transporting protein [21–23]; however, in the presence of high glucose concentrations in a dose dependent manner such as 15 or 30 mM, develop INR and GLUT 4 with glucose uptake [24]. Additionally, high glucose promotes endothelial dysfunction via excessive intracellular glucose accumulation and oxidative stress, leading to increased production proinflammatory cytokines, ROS with induction of the aldose reductase pathway and formation of advanced glycation end products (AGEs) as well as enhanced signaling of protein kinase C (PKC) and mitogen-activated protein kinases (MAPK) [8, 25]. The ROS causes acceleration of cellular growth and promotes synthesis and secretion of proinflammatory cytokines IL-6 and IL-8 which are implicated in the pathogenesis of atherosclerosis [24, 26, 27].

2. Inflammation and oxidative stress effects of glucose and fatty acids on human T-lymphocytes and HAEC

Since both hyperglycemia and hyperlipidemia are important contributing risk for cardiovascular events in diabetes and deleterious effects of hyperglycemia have been well documented in vivo and in vitro in both T-lymphocytes and HAEC [12, 15, 17, 19, 20, 28–30], we studied the effects of various fatty acids on these cells. The saturated fatty acid palmitic acid, the major fatty acid in plasma, and the monounsaturated, oleic (C18:1), polyunsaturated fatty acids, linoleic (C18:2), omega 3 fatty acid α-linolenic (C18:3), and arachidonic (C20:4) acids were used in 1, 100 and 300 uM concentrations during incubations for 0, 24, 48, 72 and 96 hours. These cells were incubated alone or with glucose concentrations of 5 mM, 15 mM and 30 mM or with a combination with linolenic acid. Unsaturated fatty acids such as linoleic, oleic, linolenic, and arachidonic acids were not able to activate these cells. These studies showed that palmitic acid, but not oleic, linoleic, linolenic or arachidonic acids, exhibited dose and time dependent responses of deleterious effects of palmitic acid by demonstrating increased levels of ROS and lipid peroxidation (malondialdehyde- MDA), emergence of receptors for insulin, IGF-1, IL-2, GLUT 4, inflammatory and proinflammatory effects detected by the emergence of interleukin (IL) cytokines IL-1B, IL-6, IL-8, IL-2, IL-10, and TNFα. and CD69 in T lymphocytes [31]. There was also increased expression of E-selectin, GLUT 4, INR, ROS, lipid peroxidation, inflammatory and proinflammatory effects detected by the emergence of interleukin (IL) cytokines IL-1B, IL-6, IL-8, IL-2, IL-10, and TNFα in the HAEC incubated with palmitic acid and/or glucose. **Table 1** shows the effects of the glucose, palmitic and linolenic incubated alone or in combination with the T lymphocytes. The omega 3 fatty acid linolenic acid had a repressive effect on the deleterious effects of the high glucose and palmitic acid. **Table 2** shows the effects of the glucose, palmitic and linolenic incubated alone or in combination with the HAEC. The omega 3 fatty acid linolenic acid had a repressive effect on the deleterious effects of the high glucose and palmitic acid in the HAEC as well.

Studies have shown that dietary SFA can induce insulin resistance [32–35]. We hypothesized that unsaturated fatty acids (UFA) may provide a protective mechanism against the prooxidant effects of hyperglycemia and high SFA such as palmitic acid. Our studies have also shown that SFA palmitic acid induces expression of GPR40 and FATCD/36 involved in inflammation and the unsaturated fatty acid linolenic acid can reverse the production of these receptors in aortic endothelial cells [36].

Thus, linolenic acid may serve as a protective mechanism against the deleterious effects of high glucose and palmitate in human T-cells and HAEC and reduce the inflammatory process observed with high blood glucose and high saturated fatty acid foods as observed in diabetes, prediabetes, cardiovascular disease and other health conditions.

3. High protein and high carbohydrate diets effects on remission of prediabetes, inflammation, oxidative stress and cardiovascular risk factors

Lifestyle changes of diet and exercise can reduce the risk of developing diabetes by 58% [37]; whereas, pharmaceutical intervention reduces the risk by 32% (metformin) [37] and 72% (pioglitazone) [38]. Hyperglycemia and hyperlipidemia are important risk factors of developing diabetes and cardiovascular disease; however, no diet had been established for reducing the hyperglycemia and hyperlipidemia. Although numerous diets have been recommended for T2DM and non-diabetics [39–43], and suggested advantages of low-carbohydrate [44, 45] or high protein [46, 47] diets, there had been no consensus on a specific weight loss diet to manage blood glucose in T2DM and converting from T2DM to normal glucose tolerance. We studied the effects of macronutrients in a High Protein (HP) (30% Kcal protein,

	Glucose (G)			Palmitic acid (P)			Linolenic acid (L)			G (15 mM) + P (100 µM)	G (15 mM) + L (100 µM)	G (15 mM) + P (100 µM) + L (100 µM)
	5 mM	**15 mM**	**30 mM**	**5 µM**	**100 µM**	**300 µM**	**5 µM**	**100 µM**	**300 µM**			
Activation markers												
CD69 (%)	<1	11 ± .7*	26 ± 3*	<1	2 ± 1*	3 ± .8*	<1	<1	<1	14 ± 2†	4 ± .6†	6 ± 1.7Δ
INSR (%)	0	5 ± 1*	12 ± 2*	0	8 ± 2*	14 ± 2*	0	0	0	12 ± 2†	2 ± .6†	5 ± 2Δ
CD25 (%)	0	6 ± 1*	17 ± 3*	0	10 ± 2*	18 ± 3*	0	0	0	15 ± 3†	3 ± .5†	6.5 ± .4Δ
Oxidative stress												
DCF (%)	0	7 ± 1.2*	23 ± 2*	1 ± .3	14 ± 2*	30 ± 3*	0	0	0	21 ± 3†	4 ± .5†	8 ± 2Δ
TBA (MDA)	0	6 ± 2*	19 ± 4*	.8 ± .1	10 ± 2*	22 ± 3*	0	0	0	15 ± 2†	3 + 1†	9 ± 1Δ
Inflammation												
TNFα (pg/ml)	7 ± 1	36 ± 2*	185 ± 4*	7 ± 1	71 ± 3*	98 ± 3*	7 ± 2	8 ± 3	7 ± 2	94 ± 4†	15 ± 2†	49 ± 3Δ
IL-1β (pg/ml)	3 ± 1	18 ± *	51 ± 2*	3 ± 1	21 ± 2*	34 ± 2*	3 ± 1	4 ± 1	3 ± 1	29 ± 3†	11 ± 1†	17 ± 2Δ
IL-6 (pg/ml)	6 ± 1	43 ± 2*	171 ± 3*	6 ± 2	58 ± 3*	87 ± 3*	6 ± 2	7 ± 2	6 ± 2	128 ± 4†	27 ± 3†	71 ± 3Δ
IL-8 (pg/ml)	12 ± 2	184 ± 3*	215 ± 5*	10 ± 2	78 ± 3*	102 ± 4*	9 ± 2	9 ± 2	9 ± 2	235 ± 6†	83 ± 3†	118 ± 3Δ
IL-2 (pg/ml)	23 ± 2	69 ± 3*	172 ± 4*	23 ± 3	87 ± 4*	119 ± 3*	23 ± 2	24 ± 3	23 ± 2	153 ± 4†	36 ± 3†	89 ± 2Δ
IL-10 (pg/ml)	9 ± 1	20 ± 2*	69 ± 3*	9 ± 2	34 ± 3*	58 ± 3*	9 ± 2	9 ± 2	9 ± 2	47 ± 3†	12 ± 1†	29 ± 3Δ
Inflammation inhibition with NFkBi												
TNFα + NFkBi	6 ± 1	6 ± 1	6 ± 2	5 ± 1	5 ± 2	6 ± 2	5 ± 1	5 ± 1	5 ± 1	7 ± 2	7 ± 2	7 ± 3

Values indicate mean ± SE. Measured at 72 hours.
**P < 0.05 from baseline.*
†p < 0.05 from glucose (15 mM) or palmitate (100 uM).
Δp < 0.05 from glucose (15 mM) + palmitate (100 uM).

Table 1.
Effect of glucose, palmitic acid, and α-linolenic acid on activation of human T cells, proinflammatory cytokines and IL-10 and oxidative stress (DCF and MDA) at 72 hrs of incubation.

	Glucose (G)			Palmitic Acid (P)			Linolenic Acid (L)			G (15 mM) + P (100 μM)	G (15 mM) + L (100 μM)	G (15 mM) + P (100 μM) + L (100 μM)
	5 mM	15 mM	30 mM	5 μM	100 μM	300 μM	5 μM	100 μM	300 μM			
E-Selectin%	<1	$24 \pm 4^{*}$	$39 \pm 3^{\dagger}$	<1	$18 \pm 3^{*}$	$42 \pm 4^{\dagger}$	<1	<1	<1	$39 \pm 7^{\dagger}$	$11 \pm 3^{\dagger}$	$15 \pm 4^{\Delta}$
INSR (%)	<1	$25 \pm 3^{*}$	$37 \pm 3^{\dagger}$	<1	$8 \pm 2^{*}$	$22 \pm 3^{\dagger}$	<1	<1	<1	$30 \pm 3^{\dagger}$	$8 \pm 2^{\dagger}$	$12 \pm 2^{\Delta}$
IGF-IR %	<1	$8 \pm 2^{*}$	$20 \pm 2^{\dagger}$	<1	$10 \pm 3^{*}$	$24 \pm 3^{\dagger}$	<1	<1	<1	$16 \pm 3^{\dagger}$	$4 \pm 1^{\dagger}$	$5 \pm 2^{\Delta}$
GLUT 4%	<1	$17 \pm 3^{*}$	$34 \pm 3^{\dagger}$	<1	$3 \pm 1^{*}$	$8 \pm 2^{\dagger}$	<1	<1	<1	$22 \pm 3^{\dagger}$	$6 \pm 2^{\dagger}$	$7 \pm 2^{\Delta}$
GLUT 1%	3 ± 1	$19 \pm 3^{*}$	$30 \pm 3^{\dagger}$	3 ± 1	$6 \pm 2^{*}$	$13 \pm 3^{\dagger}$	3 ± 1	3 ± 2	3 ± 2	$21 \pm 3^{\dagger}$	$8 \pm 2^{\dagger}$	$9 \pm 2^{\Delta}$
IRS-1%	0	$15 \pm 3^{*}$	$34 \pm 3^{\dagger}$	0	$7 \pm 2^{*}$	$11 \pm 2^{\dagger}$	0	0	0	$17 \pm 3^{\dagger}$	$6 \pm 2^{\dagger}$	$8 \pm 2^{\Delta}$
Oxidative stress												
DCF (%)	0	$9 \pm 1^{*}$	$26 \pm 2^{\dagger}$	0	$14 \pm 2^{*}$	$34 \pm 4^{\dagger}$	0	0	0	$22 \pm 3^{\dagger}$	$4 \pm .5^{\dagger}$	$7 \pm 2^{\Delta}$
MDA (μM)	0	$7 \pm 2^{*}$	$20 \pm 4^{\dagger}$	0	$12 \pm 2^{*}$	$29 \pm 4^{\dagger}$	0	0	0	$17 \pm 2^{\dagger}$	$3 + 1^{\dagger}$	$8 \pm 1^{\Delta}$
Inflammatory markers												
TNFα (pg/ml)	18 ± 1	$39 \pm 2^{*}$	$172 \pm 4^{\dagger\wedge}$	18 ± 2	$23 \pm 4^{*}$	$137 \pm 5^{\dagger}$	18 ± 2	18 ± 3	19 ± 2	$94 \pm 4^{\dagger}$	$15 \pm 2^{\dagger}$	$49 \pm 3^{\Delta}$
IL-1β (pg/ml)	3 ± 1	$18 \pm 2^{*}$	$51 \pm 2^{\dagger}$	2 ± 1	$7 \pm 2^{*}$	$10 \pm 2^{\dagger}$	2 ± 1	3 ± 1	3 ± 1	$29 \pm 3^{\dagger}$	$11 \pm 1^{\dagger}$	$17 \pm 2^{\Delta}$
IL-6 (pg/ml)	21 ± 3	$36 \pm 3^{*}$	$53 \pm 4^{\dagger}$	19 ± 3	$31 \pm 4^{*}$	$66 \pm 4^{\dagger}$	17 ± 2	18 ± 3	18 ± 2	$128 \pm 4^{\dagger}$	$27 \pm 3^{\dagger}$	$71 \pm 3^{\Delta}$
IL-8 (pg/ml)	171 ± 1	$384 \pm 6^{*}$	$915 \pm 7^{\dagger}$	170±	$286 \pm 3^{*}$	$759 \pm 9^{\dagger}$	167 ± 7	169 ± 9	171 ± 8	$335 \pm 6^{\dagger}$	$203 \pm 3^{\dagger}$	$218 \pm 3^{\Delta}$
IL-2 (pg/ml)	0	0	0	0	0	0	0	0	0	0	0	0
IL-10 (pg/ml)	2 ± 1	2 ± 1	2 ± 1	2 ± 1	3 ± 1	3 ± 1	2 ± 1	2 ± 1	2 ± 1	2 ± 1	2 ± 1	2 ± 1

Values indicate mean ± SE. Measured at 72 hours.
**P < 0.05 from baseline.*
†*p < 0.05 from glucose (15 mM) or palmitate (100 uM).*
$^{\Delta}$*p < 0.05 from glucose (15 mM) + palmitate (100 uM).*

Table 2.
Effect of hyperglycemia (glucose), hyperlipidemia (palmitic acid) on activation of human aortic endothelial cells, inflammation (proinflammatory cytokines and IL-10) and oxidative stress (DCF and MDA) and the salutary effect of α-linolenic acid.

	HP (n = 12)			HC (n = 12)			
Parameters	Baseline	6 months	p*	Baseline	6 months	p*	p**
Age	35.9 ± 2.1			35.4 ± 2.0			0.8981
Ethnicity AA/C	7/5			10/2			0.3701†
BMI (kg/m^2)	41.3 ± 1.8	37.3 ± 1.9	0.0005	37.0 ± 1.5	33.5 ± 1.4	0.0005	0.5512
% Weight loss		9.8 ± 1.4	0.0005		9.3 ± 1.6	0.0005	0.9323
HOMA IR	4.0 ± 0.8	1.4 ± 0.2	0.0005	3.7 ± 0.4	2.3 ± 0.3	0.0005	0.0033
ISI (Matsuda Index)	2.7 ± 0.5	6.7 ± 0.5	0.0005	2.6 ± 0.3	3.5 ± 0.4	0.0005	<0.0001
Beta cell function	4.4 ± 0.4	11.8 ± 2.5	0.0005	4.2 ± 0.4	6.3 ± 0.6	0.0005	<0.0001
Cardiovascular risk factors							
TG (mg/dl)	107 ± 10	81 ± 2.7	0.0005	102 ± 5.7	94 ± 3.8	0.0117	0.0907
Free fatty acids (mM)	0.57 ± 0.03	0.45 ± 0.03	0.0010	0.56 ± 0.04	0.73 ± 0.07	0.0342	0.0002
hCRP (mg/L)	5.9 ± 0.2	3.8 ± 0.4	0.0005	5.8 ± 0.2	5.0 ± 0.2	0.0005	0.0003
E-selectin (ng/ml)	42.6 ± 1.5	34.0 ± 1.3	0.0005	43.4 ± 1.3	39.7 ± 1.1	0.0005	0.0007
BP (SBP/DBP)	129/ 83 ± 1.5/1.3	119/ 74 ± 1.1/1.3	0.0005/ 0.0005	128/ 82 ± 1.7/1.4	120/ 75 ± 1.7/1.0	0.0005/ 0.0005	0.1029/ 0.2579
Inflammation							
TNFα (pg/ml)	5.9 ± 1.3	4.1 ± 0.2	0.0005	6.0 ± 0.2	5.1 ± 0.1	0.0005	<0.0001
IL-6 (pg/ml)	6.2 ± 0.2	4.9 ± 0.2	0.0005	5.8 ± 0.2	5.4 ± 0.1	0.0005	<0.0001
Oxidative stress							
DCF (μM)	3.2 ± 0.1	2.4 ± 0.1	0.0005	3.2 ± 0.1	2.9 ± 0.1	0.0005	<0.0001
MDA (μM)	1.1 ± 0.06	0.7 ± 0.05	0.0005	1.1 ± 0.05	0.9 ± 0.05	0.0005	0.0004
% Compliance		94% ±1.5%			91% ± 4.8%		0.3979

Significant level for multiple comparison is set at P = 0.01.
**Indicates Wilcoxon Signed Rank Test.*
***Indicates Wilcoxon Rank Sum Test for 6 months HP vs. HC.*
†Fisher's exact test.
AA/C, African American/Caucasian; BP, blood pressure; SBP, systolic blood pressure; DBP, diastolic blood pressure; TG, triglyceride; hsCRP, high sensitivity C-reactive protein; TNF-α, tumor necrosis factor-α; IL-6, interleukin-6; DCF, dichlorofluorescein; MDA, malondialdehyde.

Table 3.
Effect of high protein or high carbohydrate diets on weight loss, insulin sensitivity, Beta cell function, markers of cardiovascular risk factors, inflammation and oxidative stress in obese premenopausal, non-diabetic women.

40% Kcal carbohydrate (CHO) and 30% Kcal fat) diet versus a High Carbohydrate (HC) (15% Kcal protein, 55% Kcal CHO and 30% Kcal fat) diet in obese, normal glucose tolerance premenopausal women [48] (see **Table 3**) and in obese prediabetic (Impaired Glucose Tolerant (IGT)) women and men [49] (see **Table 4**) in randomized, controlled clinical trials. In both studies all food was provided with weekly food pick up with daily menus and weight checks for 6 months. Although our study of IGT subjects [49] and obese, non-diabetic, women [48] had significant

	HP (n = 12)			HC (n = 12)			
Parameters	**Baseline**	**6 months**	**p***	**Baseline**	**6 months**	**p***	**p****
% Remission		100			33.3		0.001
Age	43.1 ± 1.3			41.1 ± 1.7			0.96
Ethnicity AA/C	10/2			9/3			
Female/male	9/3			10/2			
% Weight loss		9.8 ± 1.4	<0.001		11.3 ± 1.8	<0.001	0.692
BMI (kg/m^2)	40.5 ± 1.8	37.3 ± 1.9	<0.001	37.4 ± 1.7	33.8 ± 1.6	0.002	0.391
% LeanBMchange		2.6 ± 0.4	0.002		−3.0 ± 1.1	0.005	0.001
% Fat BM change		−2.5 ± 0.4	0.006		−3.5 ± 0.9	0.007	0.04
Insulin sensitivity							
HbA1c %	6.0 ± 0.015	5.46 ± 0.12	.0005	5.93 ± 0.12	5.73 ± 0.17	0.005	<0.0001
HOMA IR	4.79 ± 0.71	1.58 ± 0.38	0.0005	4.74 ± 0.72	3.34 ± 0.78	0.005	<0.0001
ISI (Matsuda index)	2.3 ± 0.3	6.5 ± 1.1	0.0005	2.3 ± 0.3	3.2 ± 0.4	0.005	0.003
Cardiovascular risk factors							
BP (SBP/DBP)	130/81 ± 3/2	116/72 ± 2/2	0.01/0.01	126/81 ± 3/2	118/74 ± 3/3	0.01/0.01	0.73/0.77
TG (mg/dl)	106.9 ± 10	69.4 ± 6.7	0.001	110.1 ± 11	98.7 ± 9.1	0.002	0.04
LDL (mg/dl)	105.9 ± 4.4	82.4 ± 3.4	0.0005	106.2 ± 5.6	101.9 ± 6.2	0.096	0.037
Cholesterol (mg/dl)	165.3 ± 5.7	151.8 ± 5.3	0.0005	167.9 ± 6.1	161.7 ± 6.3	0.02	0.42
HDL (mg/dl)	44.9 ± 1.7	46.3 ± 1.4	0.10	45.8 ± 2.6	46.2 ± 2.5	0.69	0.85
FFA (mM)	0.74 ± 0.05	0.46 ± 0.04	0.0010	0.74 ± 0.04	0.72 ± 0.05	0.064	0.0001
hCRP (mg/L)	9.1 ± 0.4	4.0 ± 0.3	0.0001	8.8 ± 0.3	6.4 ± 0.2	0.005	0.0003
E-Selectin (ng/ml)	53.7 ± 1.5	35.0 ± 1.1	0.0005	53.4 ± 1.6	44.6 ± 1.7	0.005	0.0005
Proinflammatory cytokines							
TNF-α (pg/ml)	12.8 ± 0.4	3.8 ± 0.2	0.0005	12.5 ± 0.4	9.6 ± 0.3	0.005	<0.0001
IL-6 (pg/ml)	8.57 ± 0.34	4.55 ± 0.13	0.0005	8.43 ± 0.22	6.8 ± 0.11	0.0005	<0.0001
Oxidative stress							
DCF (μM)	3.9 ± 0.2	2.5 ± 0.3	0.0004	4.0 ± 0.1	3.2 ± 0.2	0.01	<0.0001
MDA (μM)	1.5 ± 0.07	0.6 ± 0.04	0.0008	1.5 ± 0.08	1.2 ± 0.04	0.02	0.0004

*Indicates Wilcoxon Signed Rank Test for comparison of Baseline to 6 months.
**Indicates Wilcoxon Rank Sum Test for 6 months comparison of HP vs. HC.

Table 4.
Effect of HP or HC diets on remission of prediabetes, weight loss, glucose, insulin sensitivity, cardiovascular risk factors, proinflammatory cytokines and oxidative stress.

weight loss (9–10%) on the HP or HC diets, in both studies the HP diet provided greater improvement in insulin sensitivity, reduced CVR factors, decreased inflammation and inflammatory cytokines, decreased oxidative stress, decreased lipid peroxidation, adipokines markers and increased incretin responses [50, 51]. The HP

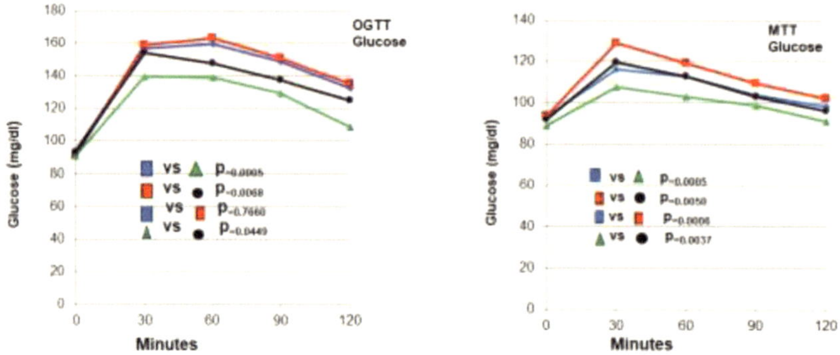

Figure 1.
Obese premenopausal non-diabetic women mean glucose values for the OGTT and MTT from 0 to 120 minutes for the ■ baseline-HP, ■ baseline-HC, ▲ 6 months-HP, and ● 6 months-HC diets for the 12 HP subjects and the 12 HC subjects. P values are the significance of area under the curve for glucose for the OGTT and MTT comparing baseline-HP with 6 month-HP, baseline-HC with 6 month-HC, baseline-HP with baseline-HC, and 6 month-HP with 6 month-HC diets.

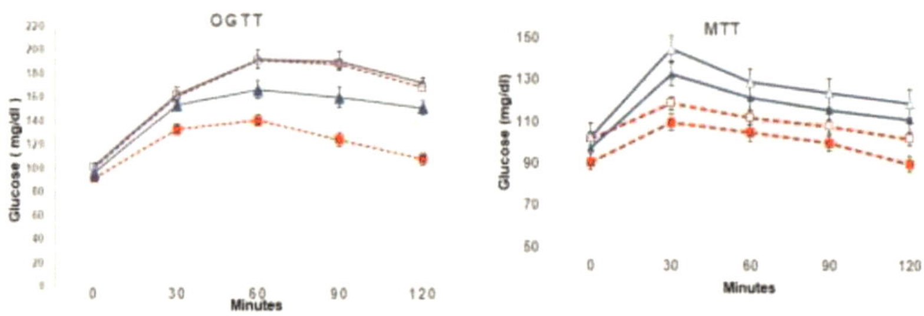

Figure 2.
This figure shows the mean ± SD of glucose for the 2 hour OGTT and MTT for the 12 HP diet subjects and the 12 HC diet subjects. The symbols represent the following: □ HP diet baseline (HP-Bl) and ■ HP diet at 6 months (HP-6 m) dotted lines. △ HC diet baseline (HC-Bl) and ▲ HC diet at 6 months (HC-6 m) solid lines. P values for the glucose AUC for the OGTT are: HP-Bl vs. HP-6 m = 0.0005; HC-Bl vs. HC-6 m = 0.005; HP-Bl vs. HC-Bl = 0.8; HP-6 m vs. HC-6 m = 0.0001. P values for the glucose AUC for the MTT are: HP-Bl vs. HP-6 m = 0.0005; HC-Bl vs. HC-6 m = 0.005; HP-Bl vs. HC-Bl = 0.01, HP-6 m vs. HC-6 m = 0.0001. AUC, area under the curve; HP, High Protein diet; HC, High Carbohydrate diet.

diet caused a smaller increase in blood glucose with the MTT compared to the HC diet MTT in both obese, normal glucose tolerance premenopausal women (see **Figure 1**) and in obese prediabetic women and men (see **Figure 2**), thereby, reducing the hyperglycemia compared to that observed with a HC meal. Lipids are considered a primary risk factor for CV disease and dietary composition can affect the lipid profile and its metabolism. Our studies showed greater decrease in triglycerides in the HP diet demonstrating that increasing the protein in the diet may alter the lipid profile in a beneficial way.

Also, the HP diet subjects had an increase in percent body muscle mass and decrease in percent fat mass at 6 months, whereas, the HC diet subjects had a decrease in percent lean and fat mass. Additionally, the HP group had an increase in their resting metabolic rate (RMR) at 6 months, and an increase in the FGF21 which may be indicative of browning of fat [52, 53]. Epigenetic DNA methylation data showed a change in the methylation with remission of prediabetes in the areas of metabolism, cancer and heart related genes [54, 55].

It has been shown that protein intake by itself induces insulin release and is different in diabetic and non-diabetic individuals [56]. Our study showed a lower insulin response to the HP than the HC diet in both studies. This suggests that HP diets may help preserve the Beta cells by increasing sensitivity and decreasing insulin load per meal. Our studies on the incretin response to HP and HC diets showed an increased release in GLP-1 and GIP with the HP diet compared to the HC diet [57]. Treatment of T2DM subjects with GLP-1 receptor agonists and DPP-4 inhibitors have been found to improve insulin sensitivity [58, 59]. This suggests that our HP diet may be beneficial in treating T2DM and have cardiovascular benefits.

This prompted us to study the effect of the HP and HC diets on remission of T2DM. Our current randomized clinical trial of Remission of Type 2 Diabetes to normal glucose tolerance (NGT) comparing a HP diet to a HC diet has demonstrated a 100% remission of Type 2 Diabetic subjects to normal glucose tolerance who were diagnosed with the past 2 years and were randomized to the HP diet for 6 months.

However, the HC diet was not very effective with only one subject having remission to normal glucose tolerance. T2D adults aged 20–65 years were randomized to a HP or HC diet for 6 months with all food provided. Caloric need for weight loss was determined by Resting Metabolic Rate (RMR) -500 calories/day. Oral Glucose Tolerance Tests (OGTT) were performed at Baseline and 6 months to determine T2D/NGT status. A Baseline glucose ≥126 mg/dl and HbA1c ≥ 6.5% and 2 hr. glucose >199 mg/dl was considered T2D and remission was a baseline glucose <126 mg/ml and HbA1c < 6.5% and 2 hr. glucose <140 mg/dl. DXA was done at baseline and 6 months to determine bone, lean and fat mass. Food pick up and menus were provided weekly for 6 months along with and weekly weight checks. The T2D subjects on HP diet had 100% remission to NGT while the HC diet subjects had 33% remission. Both diet groups had significant weight loss (HP =15.4 ± 5 lb., HC = 19.9 ± 5 lb), improvement in insulin sensitivity determined by HOMA IR [HP (BL 5.3 ± 0.29; 6 months 2.1 ± 0.13)], [HC (BL 5.2 ± 0.27; 6 months 4.4 ± 0.26)] and decrease in HbA1c [HP (BL 7.7 ± .05; 6 mo 5.6 ± .02)], [HC (BL 7.8 ± .04; 6 mo 6.6 ± .06)] and blood pressure improvement S/D [HP (BL 129/85, 6 months 117/78)], [HC (BL 130/85; 6 months 117/78)]. The HP group had a 2.7% ± 0.4% increase in lean body mass and 2.9 ± 0.4% decrease in fat mass while the HC group had a 1.9% ± 0.3 and 3.3 ± 0.9% decrease in lean and fat mass, respectively. The HP diet provided greater improvement in insulin sensitivity, reduced CVR factors, decreased inflammation and inflammatory cytokines, decreased oxidative stress, decreased lipid peroxidation, adipokines markers and increased incretin responses than the HC diet. Both diets resulted in weight loss, improvement in glucose tolerance and insulin sensitivity but only the HP diet produced 100% remission of T2D to NGT [60].

4. Discussion

High glucose levels initiates inflammatory markers, ROS and hyperglycemia induced pathways in both T lymphocytes and HAEC. Hyperglycemia induced pathways of endothelial damage can activate ERK1/2MAPK cascade via PKC or Advanced Glycation End (AGE) products [4, 25]. High glucose can induce formation of AGE products which are proteins or lipids which become glycated due to exposure to glucose. These AGE products are implicated in aging and many degenerative diseases such as diabetes, atherosclerosis, kidney disease and possibly Alzheimer's disease [61–67]. The glycation of various protein and lipids causes improper function of these molecules, for example, inactivation of anti-aging genes critical to prevent hyperglycemia and hyperlipidemia induced inflammation [68, 69]. We have shown that with remission of prediabetes and better glucose control numerous genes have changes in DNA methylation affecting gene

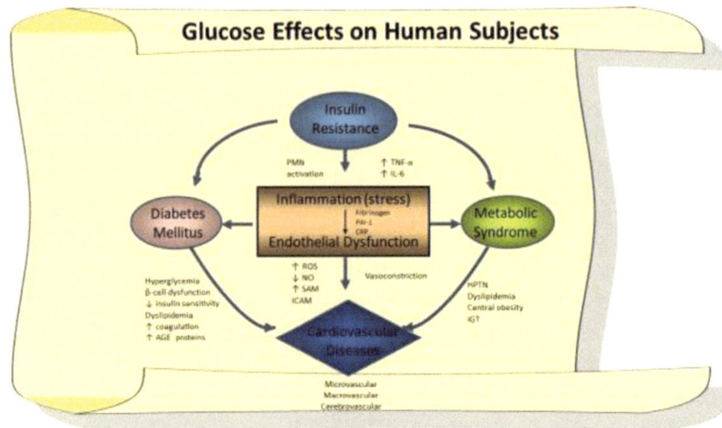

Figure 3.
This figure shows the relationship and effects of high glucose and lipids (dyslipidemia) on inflammation, cardiovascular disease, insulin resistance, diabetes mellitus and metabolic syndrome.

expression and translation of which any of these genes are involved in insulin signaling, cardiovascular disease and inflammation [55]. The effects of hyperglycemia and hyperlipidemia we have shown on the T-lymphocytes will affect the immune system and its function as well as the endothelial cells involved in cardiovascular function. The decrease in inflammation with the decrease in blood glucose and lipids in subjects with the HP diet correlates with the effects of glucose and fatty acids on inflammation and oxidative stress we observed in the in vitro studies of the T-lymphocytes and aortic endothelial cells. This demonstrates the effects of the high glucose and lipids on cells and the whole body. Thus, indicating the importance of good glucose control in diabetic subjects as well as prediabetic and normal subjects to prevent the inflammatory response. **Figure 3** is a diagram of the effects of high glucose on cells and tissues which can be controlled with normal glucose and free fatty acids.

Our previous studies of subjects with Adult Respiratory Distress Syndrome (ARDS) showed the high levels of inflammatory markers. [70, 71]. Reports from the CDC show the deleterious effects COVID-19 has on diabetic subjects indicating that the combined inflammation of the virus plus the high inflammatory markers in diabetic subjects is very detrimental to the subjects. Thus, good glucose control could help decrease the high inflammatory markers observed with the COVID-19.

5. Conclusions

Approximately 65% of patients with T2DM die as a result of cardiovascular disease with hyperglycemia and hyperlipidemia being important risk factors for cardiovascular diseases. Both Type 2 diabetes (T2DM) and atherosclerosis are considered to be inflammatory processes. Human T-lymphocytes (T-cells) and Human Aortic Endothelial cells (HAEC) have been shown to be components of plaque formation in atherosclerosis. T cells and HAEC are unique in that in their naive state they have no insulin receptors responsive to insulin but become activated in the presence of in vitro and in situ hyperglycemic conditions such as diabetic and/or hyperlipidemia of saturated fatty acids (SFA). The unsaturated fatty acid (UFA) α-linolenic acid partially inhibits the activation of T cells induced by either glucose or SFA palmitate alone or in combination. Thus, linolenic acid may serve as a protective mechanism against the deleterious effects of high glucose and SFAs in human T-cells and reduce the inflammatory process observed with high blood glucose and high saturated fatty acid foods.

A diet which causes a lower blood glucose and lipids after ingestion is beneficial in controlling glucose and lipids as we have shown with the High Protein Diet. The HP diet resulted in 100% remission of pre-diabetes to normal glucose tolerance while the HC diet resulted in only 33% remission. These results show that high efficacy can be achieved with dietary modification if parameters are rigorously controlled and monitored. The HP group had greater improvement in insulin sensitivity, greater reduction in CVR factors, oxidative stress (ROS) and inflammation than the HC diet group. The HP diet prediabetes group percent lean body mass (LM) increased while percent body FM was decreased; whereas, the HC diet group lost both percent LM and FM. Since all subjects were minimally physically active and there was no physical activity modification during the 6 months on the diets, we were able to study the direct effect of the HP versus HC diets. The HC group sustained higher glucose and insulin levels with both the OGTTs and MTTs compared with the HP diet group after 6 months on the diet. The greater insulin response with the HC diet likely equates to greater stress on β cells. The higher sustained glucose elevation with ingestion of glucose or higher glycemic foods as in the HC diet correlates with increased oxidative stress and inflammation in the HC group compared with the HP group. Antioxidant enzymes induced by repeated intake of excess energy in the form of high-fat, HC diets are not sufficient to block oxidative stress and inflammation in healthy human subjects [72]. Thus, the fact that our HP diet had a significantly greater reduction in blood glucose, free fatty acids, ROS and inflammation markers than the HC diet in prediabetes and normal subjects demonstrates the importance of maintaining good glucose control and is of great health importance.

Author details

Frankie B. Stentz
Division of Endocrinology, Diabetes and Metabolism, Department of Medicine, The University of Tennessee Health Science Center, Memphis, TN, USA

*Address all correspondence to: fstentz@uthsc.edu

References

[1] (CDC) CfDC. National Diabetes Statistics Report, 2018. *wwwcdcgov/diabetes/data/statistics/2018StatisticsReport*. 2018.

[2] DCCT. The Effect of Intensive Treatment of Diabetes on the Development and Progression of Long-Term Complications in Insulin-Dependent Diabetes Melllitus. *N Engl J Med*. 1993;329(977–86.

[3] Haffner S. Epidemiological Studeis on the Effects of Hyperglycemia and Improvement of Glycemic Control on Macrovascular Events in Type 2 Diabetes. *Diabetes Care*. 1999;22(3):C54-C6.

[4] Stern M. Natural History of Macrovascular Disease in Type 2 Diabetes. Role of Insulin Resistance. *Diabetes Care*. 1999;22(3):C2-C5.

[5] Haffner S. Hyperglycemia as a Cardiovascular Risk Factor. *Am J Med*. 2003;115(Suppl 8A):6S–11S.

[6] (UKPDS) UPDSG. Intensive Blood-Glucose Control with Sulphonylureas or Insulin Compared with Convenional Treatment, and Risk of Complications in Patients with Type 2 Diabetes (UKPDS 33). *Lancet Diabetes Endocrinol*. 1998;352 (837–53.

[7] Kitabchi AE, Umpierrez GE, Fisher JN, Murphy MB, and Stentz FB. Thirty years of personal experience in hyperglycemic crises: diabetic ketoacidosis and hyperglycemic hyperosmolar state. *J Clin Endocrinol Metab*. 2008;93(5):1541–52.

[8] Creager M. Diabetes and Vascular DIsease: Pathophysiology, Clinical Consequences, and Medical Therapy: Part 1. *Circulation*. 2003;108(1527–32.

[9] Dandona P, Aljada A, Chaudhuri A, and Mohanty P. Endothelial dysfunction, inflammation and diabetes. *Rev Endocr Metab Disord*. 2004;5(3): 189–97.

[10] Hink U, Li H, Mollnau H, Oelze M, Matheis E, Hartmann M, Skatchkov M, Thaiss F, Stahl RA, Warnholtz A, et al. Mechanisms underlying endothelial dysfunction in diabetes mellitus. *Circ Res*. 2001;88(2):E14–22.

[11] Schnyder B, Pittet M, Durand J, and Schnyder-Candrian S. Rapid effects of glucose on the insulin signaling of endothelial NO generation and epithelial Na transport. *Am J Physiol Endocrinol Metab*. 2002;282(1):E87–94.

[12] Stentz FB, Umpierrez GE, Cuervo R, and Kitabchi AE. Proinflammatory cytokines, markers of cardiovascular risks, oxidative stress, and lipid peroxidation in patients with hyperglycemic crises. *Diabetes*. 2004;53 (8):2079–86.

[13] Ross R. Atherosclerosis–an inflammatory disease. *N Engl J Med*. 1999;340(2):115–26.

[14] Helderman JH. Role of insulin in the intermediary metabolism of the activated thymic-derived lymphocyte. *J Clin Invest*. 1981;67(6):1636–42.

[15] Stentz FB, and Kitabchi AE. De novo emergence of growth factor receptors in activated human CD4+ and CD8+ T lymphocytes. *Metabolism*. 2004;53(1): 117–22.

[16] Stentz FB, and Kitabchi AE. Activated T lymphocytes in Type 2 diabetes: implications from in vitro studies. *Curr Drug Targets*. 2003;4(6): 493–503.

[17] Stentz FB, and Kitabchi AE. Hyperglycemia-induced activation of human T-lymphocytes with de novo emergence of insulin receptors and generation of reactive oxygen species.

Biochem Biophys Res Commun. 2005;335 (2):491–5.

[18] Stentz FB, and Kitabchi AE. Palmitic acid-induced activation of human T-lymphocytes and aortic endothelial cells with production of insulin receptors, reactive oxygen species, cytokines, and lipid peroxidation. *Biochem Biophys Res Commun.* 2006;346(3):721–6.

[19] Stentz FB, and Kitabchi AE. Transcriptome and proteome expression in activated human CD4 and CD8 T-lymphocytes. *Biochem Biophys Res Commun.* 2004;324(2):692–6.

[20] Kitabchi AE, Stentz FB, and Umpierrez GE. Diabetic ketoacidosis induces in vivo activation of human T-lymphocytes. *Biochem Biophys Res Commun.* 2004;315(2):404–7.

[21] Bar RS, Boes M, Dake BL, Booth BA, Henley SA, and Sandra A. Insulin, insulin-like growth factors, and vascular endothelium. *Am J Med.* 1988;85(5A): 59–70.

[22] Chisalita SI, and Arnqvist HJ. Insulin-like growth factor I receptors are more abundant than insulin receptors in human micro- and macrovascular endothelial cells. *Am J Physiol Endocrinol Metab.* 2004;286(6):E896–901.

[23] Kaiser N, Sasson S, Feener EP, Boukobza-Vardi N, Higashi S, Moller DE, Davidheiser S, Przybylski RJ, and King GL. Differential regulation of glucose transport and transporters by glucose in vascular endothelial and smooth muscle cells. *Diabetes.* 1993;42(1):80–9.

[24] Gosmanov AR, Stentz FB, and Kitabchi AE. De novo emergence of insulin-stimulated glucose uptake in human aortic endothelial cells incubated with high glucose. *Am J Physiol Endocrinol Metab.* 2006;290(3):E516–22.

[25] Sheetz MJ, and King GL. Molecular understanding of hyperglycemia's adverse effects for diabetic complications. *JAMA.* 2002;288(20): 2579–88.

[26] Srinivasan S, Hatley ME, Reilly KB, Danziger EC, and Hedrick CC. Modulation of PPARalpha expression and inflammatory interleukin-6 production by chronic glucose increases monocyte/endothelial adhesion. *Arterioscler Thromb Vasc Biol.* 2004;24 (5):851–7.

[27] Aljada A, Ghanim H, Assian E, and Dandona P. Tumor necrosis factor-alpha inhibits insulin-induced increase in endothelial nitric oxide synthase and reduces insulin receptor content and phosphorylation in human aortic endothelial cells. *Metabolism.* 2002;51 (4):487–91.

[28] Stentz FB, and Kitabchi AE. Transcriptome and proteome expressions involved in insulin resistance in muscle and activated T-lymphocytes of patients with type 2 diabetes. *Genomics Proteomics Bioinformatics.* 2007;5(3–4):216–35.

[29] Williams SB, Goldfine AB, Timimi FK, Ting HH, Roddy MA, Simonson DC, and Creager MA. Acute hyperglycemia attenuates endothelium-dependent vasodilation in humans in vivo. *Circulation.* 1998;97(17):1695–701.

[30] Vaidyula VR, Rao AK, Mozzoli M, Homko C, Cheung P, and Boden G. Effects of hyperglycemia and hyperinsulinemia on circulating tissue factor procoagulant activity and platelet CD40 ligand. *Diabetes.* 2006;55(1):202–8.

[31] Stentz FB, Eastman, A., Christman, J.V. Hyperglycemia and Hyperlipidemia Induced Inflammation and Oxidative Stress in Human T Lymphocytes and Salutary Effects of ω- 3 Fatty Acid. *SunKrist J Diabet Clin Care.* 2020;1(1–9.

[32] Grundy SM, and Denke MA. Dietary influences on serum lipids and

lipoproteins. *J Lipid Res.* 1990;31(7): 1149–72.

[33] Roden M, Price TB, Perseghin G, Petersen KF, Rothman DL, Cline GW, and Shulman GI. Mechanism of free fatty acid-induced insulin resistance in humans. *J Clin Invest.* 1996;97(12):2859–65.

[34] Boden G. Role of fatty acids in the pathogenesis of insulin resistance and NIDDM. *Diabetes.* 1997;46(1):3–10.

[35] Koska J, Ozias MK, Deer J, Kurtz J, Salbe AD, Harman SM, and Reaven PD. A human model of dietary saturated fatty acid induced insulin resistance. *Metabolism.* 2016;65(11):1621–8.

[36] Stentz FB. AA, Kitabchi AE. . Effect of Saturated Fatty Acids and Unsaturated Fatty Acids on Fatty Acid Receptors and Transport Proteins in Aortic Endothelial Cells. *J Investig Med.* 2008;56(359.

[37] Diabetes Prevention Program. The Diabetes Prevention Program (DPP) Research Group. Reduction in the incidence of Type 2 Diabetes with lifestyle intervention or metformin. *NEJM.* 2002;346(393–403.

[38] DeFronzo RA, Tripathy D, Schwenke DC, Banerji M, Bray GA, Buchanan TA, Clement SC, Henry RR, Hodis HN, Kitabchi AE, et al. Pioglitazone for diabetes prevention in impaired glucose tolerance. *N Engl J Med.* 2011;364(12):1104–15.

[39] Franz MJ, Powers MA, Leontos C, Holzmeister LA, Kulkarni K, Monk A, Wedel N, and Gradwell E. The evidence for medical nutrition therapy for type 1 and type 2 diabetes in adults. *J Am Diet Assoc.* 2010;110(12):1852–89.

[40] Larsen RN, Mann NJ, Maclean E, and Shaw JE. The effect of high-protein, low-carbohydrate diets in the treatment of type 2 diabetes: a 12 month randomised controlled trial. *Diabetologia.* 2011;54(4):731–40.

[41] Alford BB, Blankenship AC, and Hagen RD. The effects of variations in carbohydrate, protein, and fat content of the diet upon weight loss, blood values, and nutrient intake of adult obese women. *J Am Diet Assoc.* 1990;90 (4):534–40.

[42] McManus K, Antinoro L, and Sacks F. A randomized controlled trial of a moderate-fat, low-energy diet compared with a low fat, low-energy diet for weight loss in overweight adults. *Int J Obes Relat Metab Disord.* 2001;25 (10):1503–11.

[43] Larsen TM, Dalskov SM, van Baak M, Jebb SA, Papadaki A, Pfeiffer AF, Martinez JA, Handjieva-Darlenska T, Kunesova M, Pihlsgard M, et al. Diets with high or low protein content and glycemic index for weight-loss maintenance. *N Engl J Med.* 2010; 363(22):2102–13.

[44] Nordmann AJ, Nordmann A, Briel M, Keller U, Yancy WS, Jr., Brehm BJ, and Bucher HC. Effects of low-carbohydrate vs low-fat diets on weight loss and cardiovascular risk factors: a meta-analysis of randomized controlled trials. *Arch Intern Med.* 2006; 166(3):285–93.

[45] Boden G, Sargrad K, Homko C, Mozzoli M, and Stein TP. Effect of a low-carbohydrate diet on appetite, blood glucose levels, and insulin resistance in obese patients with type 2 diabetes. *Ann Intern Med.* 2005;142(6): 403–11.

[46] Eisenstein J, Roberts SB, Dallal G, and Saltzman E. High-protein weight-loss diets: are they safe and do they work? A review of the experimental and epidemiologic data. *Nutr Rev.* 2002;60(7 Pt 1):189–200.

[47] Bray GA, Smith, S.R., de Jonge, L. Effect of dietary protein content on weight gain, energy expenditure, and body composition during overeating: a

randomized controlled trial. *JAMA.* 2012;307(1):47–55.

[48] Kitabchi AE, Stentz FB, McDaniel KA, Wan JY, Nyenwe E, and Sands CW. Effects of high-protein versus high-carbohydrate diets on markers of beta-cell function, oxidative stress, lipid peroxidation, proinflammatory cytokines, and adipokines in obese, premenopausal women without diabetes: a randomized controlled trial. *Diabetes Care.* 2013;36 (7):1919–25.

[49] Stentz FB, Brewer A, Wan J, Garber C, Daniels B, Sands C, and Kitabchi AE. Remission of pre-diabetes to normal glucose tolerance in obese adults with high protein versus high carbohydrate diet: randomized control trial. *BMJ Open Diabetes Res Care.* 2016;4 (1):e000258.

[50] Stentz F, Kimeish, O, Kitabchi, A. Effect of High Protein vs High Carbohydrate Diets on Incretins, Satiety and Cardiovascular Factors. *Diabetes.* 2014;62: (Suppl 1):1825.

[51] Stentz FB, Ammons, A. , Sands, C. Incretin and Cardiovascular Effects of Weight Loss and Remission of Prediabetes. *Diabetes.* 2018;67(Suppl 1): 544.

[52] Daniels B, Stentz, FB. Efect of Diet Composition on Remission of Prediabetes and Metabolic Parameters. *J Investig Med.* 2016;65(2):501.

[53] Fisher FM, Kleiner S, Douris N, Fox EC, Mepani RJ, Verdeguer F, Wu J, Kharitonenkov A, Flier JS, Maratos-Flier E, et al. FGF21 regulates PGC-1alpha and browning of white adipose tissues in adaptive thermogenesis. *Genes Dev.* 2012;26(3):271–81.

[54] Stentz F, Garber, C., Kitabchi, A, . Efficacy of High Protein vs. High Carbohydrate Diet on Remission of Impaired Glucose Tolerance (IGT) to Normal Glucose Tolerance (NGT). *Diabetes.* 2015;64(Supppl 1):512.

[55] Stentz FB, Patel, D. Epigenetic Changes in DNA Methylation with Remission of Prediabetes. *Diabetes.* 2017;66(1):85.

[56] Nuttall FQ, Mooradian AD, Gannon MC, Billington C, and Krezowski P. Effect of protein ingestion on the glucose and insulin response to a standardized oral glucose load. *Diabetes Care.* 1984;7(5):465–70.

[57] Stentz FB, Mikhael, A., Kineish, O, Christman, J.V, Sands, C. Incretins and Cardiovascular Effects of Weight Loss and Remission of Prediabetes. *J Diabet Clin Studies (JDCS).* 2020.

[58] American Diabetes Association. Standard of Medical Care in Diabetes. *Diabetes Care.* 2018;41(Suppl 1):S1-S7.

[59] Eng C, Kramer CK, Zinman B, and Retnakaran R. Glucagon-like peptide-1 receptor agonist and basal insulin combination treatment for the management of type 2 diabetes: a systematic review and meta-analysis. *Lancet.* 2014;384(9961):2228–34.

[60] Stentz FB, Tucker, S. , Sands, C. Remision of Type 2 Diabetes and Improvement of Metabolic Factors with a High Protein Diet *Diabetes.* 2020; Diabetes website(1862.

[61] Goldin A, Beckman JA, Schmidt AM, and Creager MA. Advanced glycation end products: sparking the development of diabetic vascular injury. *Circulation.* 2006;114 (6):597–605.

[62] Vistoli G, De Maddis D, Cipak A, Zarkovic N, Carini M, and Aldini G. Advanced glycoxidation and lipoxidation end products (AGEs and ALEs): an overview of their mechanisms of formation. *Free Radic Res.* 2013;47 Suppl 1(3–27.

[63] Chaudhuri J, Bains Y, Guha S, Kahn A, Hall D, Bose N, Gugliucci A, and Kapahi P. The Role of Advanced Glycation End Products in Aging and Metabolic Diseases: Bridging Association and Causality. *Cell Metab.* 2018;28(3):337–52.

[64] Yan SF, D'Agati V, Schmidt AM, and Ramasamy R. Receptor for Advanced Glycation Endproducts (RAGE): a formidable force in the pathogenesis of the cardiovascular complications of diabetes & aging. *Curr Mol Med.* 2007;7(8):699–710.

[65] Brownlee M. The pathobiology of diabetic complications: a unifying mechanism. *Diabetes.* 2005;54(6):1615–25.

[66] Prasad A, Bekker P, and Tsimikas S. Advanced glycation end products and diabetic cardiovascular disease. *Cardiol Rev.* 2012;20(4):177–83.

[67] Srikanth V, Maczurek A, Phan T, Steele M, Westcott B, Juskiw D, and Munch G. Advanced glycation endproducts and their receptor RAGE in Alzheimer's disease. *Neurobiol Aging.* 2011;32(5):763–77.

[68] Martins IJ. Anti-Aging Genes Improve Appetite Regulation and Reverse Cell Senescence and Apoptosis in Global Populations. *Advances in Aging Research.* 2016;5(9–26.

[69] Martins IJ. Single Gene Inactivation with Implications to Diabetes and Multiple Organ Dysfunction Symdrome. *J Clin Epigenet.* 2017;3(3–24.

[70] Stentz F, Headley, S., Tolley, E., Meduri, G.U.,. The Interaction of Proinflammatory Cytokines (PIC) and NF-kB in Acute Respiratory Distress Syndrome (ARDS) and Response to Treatment with Methylprednisolone (MP). *First International Congress on Cytokines/Chemokines in Infectious Diseases.* 1999;Bethesda, MD(American Association of Immunologists).

[71] Meduri GU, Tolley EA, Chrousos GP, and Stentz F. Prolonged methylprednisolone treatment suppresses systemic inflammation in patients with unresolving acute respiratory distress syndrome: evidence for inadequate endogenous glucocorticoid secretion and inflammation-induced immune cell resistance to glucocorticoids. *Am J Respir Crit Care Med.* 2002;165(7):983–91.

[72] Lim S, Won H, Kim Y, Jang M, Jyothi KR, Dandona P, Ha J, and Kim SS. Antioxidant enzymes induced by repeated intake of excess energy in the form of high-fat, high-carbohydrate meals are not sufficient to block oxidative stress in healthy lean individuals. *Br J Nutr.* 2011;106(10): 1544–51.

Chapter 6

Gain or Loss? The Effect of Ad Framing on the Intention to Control Sugar Intake

Kang Li

Abstract

Health authorities have pointed out that high sugar intake can cause many health problems. The aim of this research is to examine the effectiveness of ad framing (gain vs. loss vs. neither gain nor loss) on persuading people to control their sugar intake. The results of an online experiment showed that both gain and loss frame were more effective than the neutral frame. Gain frame was the most effective one to persuade people to lower sugar intake. Moreover, individual difference of regulatory focus moderated the effect of ad framing (gain vs. loss). In addition, processing fluency mediated the effects of ad framing (gain vs. neutral/loss vs. neutral) on people's intention to limit sugar intake. Contributions and implications to advertising on sugar control are discussed.

Keywords: ad framing, gain vs. loss vs. neither gain nor loss framing, regulatory focus, regulatory focus theory, processing fluency, structural equation modeling (SEM)

1. Introduction

High sugar consumption is becoming a serious problem that threats public health in many countries. Excessive sugar intake can cause a series of health consequences, such as tooth decay, obesity, diabetes, and heart diseases [1]. These health problems greatly increase the expenditure on healthcare. In the United States, one trillion dollars are spent on healthcare each year due to the national addiction to sugar [2].

The World Health Organization (WHO) is urging people to reduce the amount of sugar they eat, suggesting restriction of added sugar to less than 5% of one's dietary intake [3]. However, it is not easy for people to control sugar intake because sugar is added to so many foods in the market [3]. Given the reality of added sugar in the market, WHO suggests that people should change eating behaviors, rather than waiting for the reformulation of products [3]. Thus, it is urgent to develop effective messages to persuade people to reduce their sugar consumptions.

This study aimed at examining the effectiveness of advertising on people's intention to limit sugar intake. Specifically, three types of message framing were investigated in this study: gain-framed ads, loss-framed ads, neither gain- nor loss-framed ads.

Gain vs. loss frame is a common approach in health message design (e.g., [4, 5]). Gain frame usually emphasizes the positive results if an individual adopts a recommended behavior, while loss frame stresses the negative consequences if someone does not adopt a recommended behavior. A large amount of research in health communication has suggested that gain vs. loss frame can influence people's preferences of whether or not to adopt a health behavior. However, most health-related research focuses on behaviors related to smoking, drinking, or fitness; little research investigates the impacts of gain vs. loss framing on changing behaviors regarding sugar intake. One contribution of the current study is to fill this gap by applying message framing in the advertising of limited sugar intake and examining the effects of gain vs. loss framing in this specific health context.

Moreover, neutral framing (neither gain- nor loss-framing) has been seldom examined in the previous research. The current research included neutral framing that only presented the neutral information about sugar but emphasized neither loss nor gain in order to fully examine the effects of message framing.

Although the effects of message framing (gain vs. loss) on people's health behaviors has been found in many studies, meta-analyses (e.g., [6–10]) have shown that gain- and loss-framed messages do not have meaningful different effects on message persuasiveness. According to the results of meta-analyses, researchers have suggested that the studies of gain vs. loss framing should be focused on potential moderators that lead to meaningful framing differences [5, 7, 11]. Following this suggestion, the current study specifically investigated the moderation effects of regulatory focus on gain- vs. loss-framing.

According to regulatory focus theory [12, 13], people mainly adopt two self-regulatory orientations: promotion focus and prevention focus. Promotion focus is based on hopes and aspirations; prevention focus is motivated by security and safety emphasizes. Research showed that positively framed promotion-focused messages were more effective for people with a promotion focus, while negatively framed prevention-focused messages were more persuasive for people with a prevention focus (e.g., [14, 15]). This is most likely because people may experience regulatory fit when a message matches their regulatory focus orientation, which in turn leads them to "feel right" and then process the message more fluently (i.e., more easily) [14, 16]. The enhanced processing fluency (i.e., the ease of processing the information) further results in better persuasiveness of the message [14].

Therefore, processing fluency may play a mediator role in the interaction effect of message framing and regulatory focus on people's behavioral intention. Nevertheless, little research investigated the abovementioned relationship. Hence, another expected contribution of this study was to fill the research gaps by examining a mediated moderation relationship between regulatory focus and processing fluency in influencing the effectiveness of gain- vs. loss-framing in the context of promoting less sugar intake.

2. Literature review and theoretical framework

2.1 Gain vs. loss framing on health issues

Health professionals often attempt to maximize the impact of a health message on people's attitudes and behaviors by framing the message in different ways [17]. Gain-framed health information stresses the benefits of taking a health action, while loss-framed information emphasizes the costs of failing to engage in that action. It is necessary to note that a gain-framed message can stress the benefits by presenting either positive results that will happen or negative consequences that will not happen, whereas a loss-framed message can present either negative consequences that will happen or positive results that will not happen to address the costs [17].

Rothman et al. suggested that, based on the conceptualization of prospect theory, the impact of a given frame on a behavior depends on whether the behavior is perceived as a risk-seeking or a risk-averse course of action [17]. They further proposed that people consider a behavior as safe or risky depending on how they perceive the extent to which that behavior will cause an unpleasant outcome. For example, a detection behavior of getting a mammogram can be seen as risky (i.e., a risk-seeking behavior) because it is possible to discover breast cancer; a prevention behavior of using sunscreen is relatively safe or low risk (i.e., a risk-averse behavior) because the purpose is to prevent an unpleasant outcome of skin cancer and maintain current health.

Consistent with this viewpoint, Rothman et al. argued that loss framing is more persuasive in promoting disease detection behaviors that involve perceived risk of unpleasant outcomes, whereas gain framing is more persuasive in promoting prevention behaviors that have little risk of bad outcomes [17]. This argument has been supported by a plethora of research (e.g., [18–24]).

Since lower sugar intake can be considered a preventative behavior with little risk of bad consequences, gain framing may be more persuasive than loss framing in convincing people to adopt the recommendation to limit sugar intake. In the present study, a control condition of neither gain nor loss framing was added to further examine the effects of message framing; however, little literature provides information about the different effects among three types of framing (i.e., gain, loss, and neither gain nor loss in this study). Hence, the following hypothesis is proposed for testing and a research question is raised for exploring:

H1: Gain-framed ads lead to greater intention to limit sugar intake than loss-framed ads.

RQ1: Will ads that are neither gain nor loss framed lead to different intent to reduce sugar intake than ads that are gain and loss framed (i.e., will the effect of neutral framing on sugar-reduction intention be different than the effects of gain or loss framing)?

2.2 The moderator role of regulatory focus

Previous research has identified regulatory focus is a moderator of gain and loss frames [14]. Higgins developed regulatory focus theory and posited that when people pursue certain goals, they self-regulate their behaviors according to their regulatory orientations [12]. Two kinds of regulatory orientations were proposed by Higgin: Promotion focus and prevention focus [12]. People with promotion focus tend to take actions that advance desired results, while people with prevention focus are more likely to adopt actions that avoid undesired results.

The promotion orientation is associated with aspirations and advancement, while the prevention orientation is associated with responsibilities and safety [25]. Thus, promotion-focused people tend to approach pleasure and positive outcomes; prevention-focused people tend to avoid pain and negative outcomes [12]. Cesario, Higgins, and Scholer claimed that promotion focus and prevention focus are present in every individual to some degree because both nurturance and security are necessary survival needs [26]. However, people may have a predominant focus due to chronic individual differences, and additionally, situational features can momentarily activate one focus or the other [26].

Regulatory focus theory also posits that there are different goal-pursuit strategies for each system [25]. It distinguishes between eager means and vigilant means [25, 26]. Eager strategic means are associated with ensuring the presence of positive outcomes or against the absence of positive outcomes; therefore, this is a natural approach for promotion focus self-regulation, which concerns advancement and accomplishment [25]. In contrast, vigilance strategies ensure the absence of negative consequences or against the presence of negative consequences; accordingly, this is a natural means for prevention focus self-regulation, which concerns safety and responsibility [25]. This can be illustrated with an example of two students with different regulatory orientations. When they want to achieve the same goal of getting a decent grade in a course, the student with a promotion-focus orientation may read extra materials beyond the required readings (i.e., an eager means) to attain a good score, whereas the student with a prevention-focus orientation may make sure to fulfill all course requirements (i.e., a vigilant means) to attain a decent grade.

Higgins argued that there is a natural fit between eager means (e.g., making sure everything goes right) and promotion-focus orientation; and there is a natural fit between vigilance means (e.g., making sure nothing goes wrong) and prevention-focus orientation [27]. The value from fit is that regulatory fit experienced by a person can increase the value of what he/she is doing [27].

When a persuasive message is designed in a way that matches audiences' regulatory focus, the audiences will feel right about the conveyed information, and regulatory fit emerges [14, 28]. Cesario et al. summarized that there are two main effects when people experience regulatory fit: First, people feel right about what they are doing during the process of goal pursuit; second, the strength of their engagement in the activity of goal pursuit can be enhanced [26].

Based upon the examination of 202 studies in a variety of topics over 13 years (1998–2010), a recent meta-analyzed study conducted by Grewal et al. also found that fit match is a way to create regulatory fit [29]. According to the discussion regarding fit match [29], gain-framed and loss-framed messages separately match people's promotion regulatory focus and prevention focus, which in turn can create regulatory fit and lead people to feel right about the message. This feeling will be further transferred into the evaluation of the message and increase the message persuasiveness [30]. Hence, from another perspective, regulatory focus moderates the persuasive effect of message framing. That is, gain- and loss-framed messages have different persuasiveness under different circumstances of regulatory focus. Therefore, the following hypotheses are proposed:

H2a: For promotion-focused individuals, gain-framed ads lead to greater intentions to limit sugar intake than loss-framed ads.

H2b: For prevention-focused individuals, loss-framed ads lead to greater intentions to limit sugar intake than gain-framed ads.

2.3 The mediator role of processing fluency

It should be noted that the moderating effects of regulatory focus on the persuasiveness of framing may be mediated by processing fluency. A great deal of research has examined the impact of fluency [14]. Processing fluency refers to the extent of ease of processing a piece of information [14]. In previous research, processing fluency is often measured by reaction time or by subjective assessment of how easy/difficult to process the information [29].

Lee and Aaker [14] summarized that research has been using various stimuli across a variety of settings to promote processing fluency, such as prior exposure (e.g., [31]), expectancy (e.g., [32]), or enhanced visual clarity (e.g., [33]). It also has been suggested that process fluency can be enhanced by regulatory fit [14, 16, 34]. The reason is that compared to a message that is regulatory nonfit, people can process the message that fits their regulatory focus more easily [16]. It also can be explained as when the information is consistent rather than inconsistent with the way people naturally think when they face issues involving both positive and negative outcomes, the information might be easier to process [14].

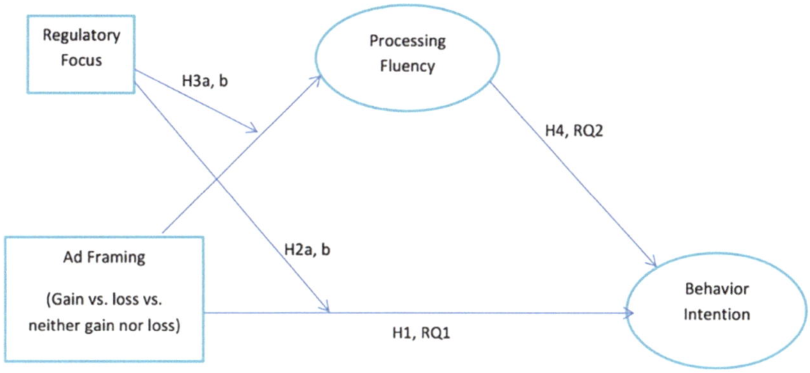

Figure 1.
Hypothesized model.

It has been suggested that processing fluency results in enhanced affective judgment [14]. People may have more favorable attitudes toward a message when they can process that message fluently [35]. Once processing fluency is enhanced, people will evaluate the message more positively, so that it will be much easier to persuade them [14, 16].

Based on the above discussion, gain and loss framing separately fits people's promotion- and prevention-focused orientation. Compared to regulatory nonfit, the regulatory fit may enhance processing fluency, and further increase the message persuasiveness. Thus, in the context of persuading people to lower their sugar intake, the following hypotheses are generated:

H3a: For promotion-focused individuals, gain-framed ads lead to greater processing fluency than loss-framed ads.

H3b: For prevention-focused individuals, loss-framed ads lead to greater processing fluency than gain-framed ads.

H4: Processing fluency mediates the interaction effects between ads' gain vs. loss framing and individuals' regulatory focus on intentions to limit sugar intake.

Since there is no literature comparing the effects of regulatory fit and processing fluency on all three types of framing (gain, loss, neither gain nor loss), the related research question is proposed to compare these effects:

RQ2: Does regulatory focus moderate three types of framing (gain, loss, neither gain nor loss) differently via processing fluency in changing people's intention to limit sugar intake?

Based on all the hypotheses and research questions, a hypothesized model is also proposed and tested in the present study (see **Figure 1**).

3. Method

3.1 Participants and procedures

This study employed a three (message framing: gain vs. loss vs. neither gain nor loss framing) × two (regulatory focus: promotion focus vs. prevention focus) between-subjects online experiment design. In the experiment, the participants completed an online survey, which contained a presentation of stimuli (six ads). The questionnaire was built and distributed via an online survey tool, Qualtrics.

The subjects were paid and recruited via an online recruiting system Amazon Mechanical Turk (MTurk). In total, there were 1,104 people who resided in the

US participated in this study. About 49% of them were female and 51% were male (544 vs. 558). They aged 18 to 74 years, with a mean age of 36.26 years (SD = 12.72). Most participants (70%) were white.

After the participants agreed with a digital consent form, they were directed to the online survey. The participants were randomly assigned into three experimental conditions (gain vs. loss vs. neither gain nor loss framing). They first answered a number of questions about their sugar-eating habits, regulatory focus orientations, and risk perceptions of excessive sugar consumption. Then they viewed an ad stimulus and responded to a following questionnaire to answer their processing fluency of viewing the ads, behavioral intention to limit sugar-eating, and demographic information.

3.2 Stimuli and measures

Six ads were designed for three experimental conditions (gain vs. loss vs. neither gain nor loss framing). Two ads were created for each condition in order to increase the external validity of the experiment: one was mainly designed by using arguments; the other one was designed by telling a personal story. All ads presented both images (e.g., a background picture with a variety of sweet snacks and beverages) and text.

The ads in the gain-framing conditions addressed the benefits of lowering sugar intake (e.g., lose weight, look younger, improve health), while the ads in the loss-framing conditions stressed the negative consequences of continuing a high-sugar diet (e.g., gain weight, look older, get diseases). In the control conditions of neither gain nor loss framing, the ads just kept neutral statements by just addressing that Americans eat too much sugar in their daily life and burning the extra calories gained from high sugar intake needs a large amount of exercise. Manipulation check was conducted, and the results showed that the stimuli ads were appropriate.

The measures of the main variables (i.e., behavioral intention, processing fluency, regulatory focus) were all drawn from the previous literature. Two control variables (i.e., sugar-eating habit, risk perception) were measured by self-created questions.

4. Results

Structural Equation Modeling (SEM) was used to explore the research questions and test the hypotheses and the model. Mplus 7 software [36] was employed to conduct the analysis. Since ad framing (gain vs. loss vs. neither gain nor loss) was a variable that had three categories, it was dummy coded into three variables in order to avoid having the analysis treat it as a continuous variable. Gain framing was first selected to be the reference group, so that the results could show the difference between gain and loss framing, as well as the difference between gain and neither gain nor loss framing. Then loss framing was chosen as the reference group for the analysis in order to compare the difference between loss framing and neither gain nor loss framing. The results showed that the model fit the data well, $\chi 2$ (18) = 32.872, $p < .05$; CFI = .995; TLI = .991; RMSEA = .027.

The results of the direct effects of ad framing (gain vs. loss vs. neither gain nor loss) on behavioral intention showed that gain framing is significantly more effective than loss framing in leading to greater intention to limit sugar intake, $\gamma = -.09$, $p < .05$. Therefore, Hypothesis 1 was supported.

For the Research Question 1, the results showed that gain framing was not only more effective than loss framing but was also significantly more effective than neither gain nor loss framing in changing behavioral intention, $\gamma = -.16, p < .001$. Moreover, loss framing was also significantly more effective than neither gain nor loss framing in changing behavioral intention, $\gamma = -.07, p < .05$.

Individuals' regulatory focus (prevention vs. promotion) was found to moderate the effect of ad framing (gain vs. loss) on behavioral intention, $\gamma = .12, p < .01$. Specifically, for promotion-focused individuals, gain framing was more effective to lead to greater intentions to limit sugar intake than loss framing; for prevention-focused individuals, loss framing was more effective than gain framing. Thus, both Hypotheses 2a and 2b were supported.

The results showed that there was no interaction effect between ad framing (gain vs. loss) and regulatory focus on processing fluency ($\gamma = .02, p = .49$). Thus, the data were not consistent with Hypotheses 3a and 3b. This finding also indicated that there was no moderated mediation among these three variables. Moreover, the indirect effect of the above tested interaction on behavioral intention through processing fluency was also not significant ($\gamma = .01, p = .60$), which confirmed that there were no moderated mediation effects among ad framing (gain vs. loss), regulatory focus, and processing fluency on behavioral intention. Thus, the data were also not consistent with Hypothesis 4.

For Research Question 2, the results showed that the interaction effects between other types of ad framing and regulatory focus on behavioral intention were also not significantly mediated by processing fluency. That is, there were no moderated mediation effects among the tested ad framing, regulatory focus, and processing fluency on behavioral intention.

However, based on the results of SEM analysis, it was found several additional findings. First, the results showed that regulatory focus not only had a significantly direct effect on behavioral intention to limit sugar intake ($\gamma = -.20, p < .001$), but also had a significantly effect on processing fluency, $\gamma = -.18, p < .01$. Promotion-focused individuals processed the ads more fluently and had greater intentions to limit sugar intake than prevention-focused individuals.

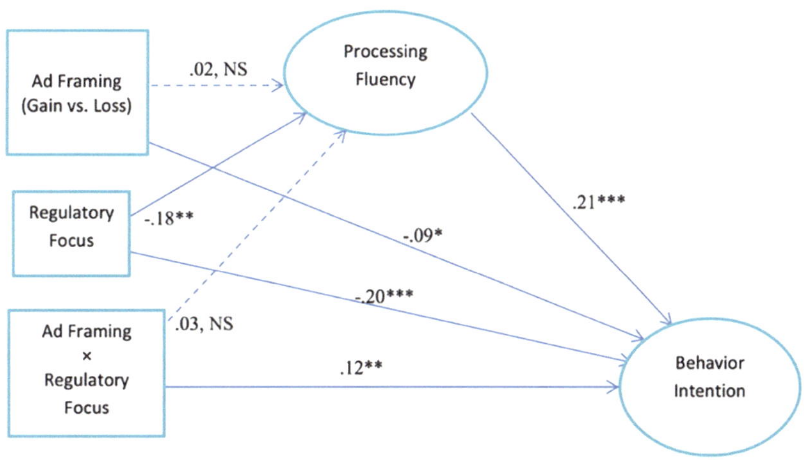

Figure 2.
*Final model (ad framing: Gain vs. loss). Note: 1. $\chi 2$ (18) = 32.872, p < .05; CFI = .995; TLI = .991; RMSEA = .027. 2. The model was evaluated by using gain framing as the reference group. 3. * indicates p < .05, ** indicates p < .01, *** indicates p < .001. 4. Dotted line indicates the effect is not statistically significant at 95% level of confidence. 5. The indirect effect of regulatory focus on behavioral intention through processing fluency is −.04, p < .01.*

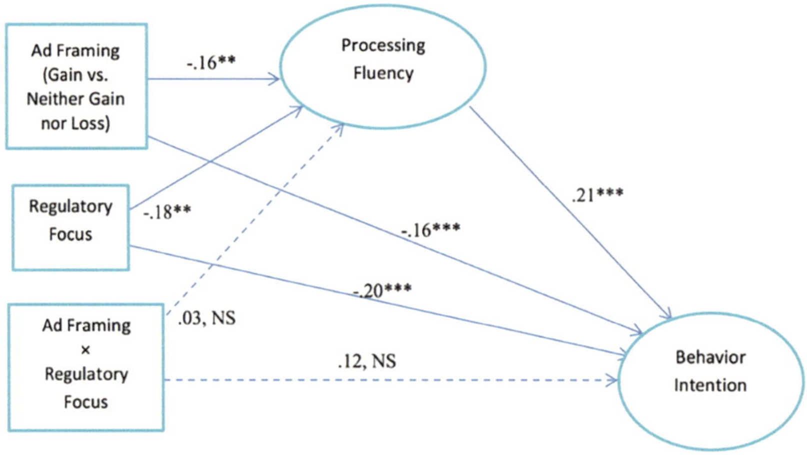

Figure 3.
*Final model (ad framing: Gain vs. neither gain nor loss). Note: 1. χ2 (18) = 32.872, p < .05; CFI = .995; TLI = .991; RMSEA = .027. 2. The model was evaluated by using gain framing as the reference group. 3. * indicates p < .05, ** indicates p < .01, *** indicates p < .001. 4. Dotted line indicates the effect is not statistically significant at 95% level of confidence. 5. The indirect effect of gain vs. neither gain nor loss framing on behavioral intention through processing fluency is −.03, p < .01. 6. The indirect effect of regulatory focus on behavioral intention through processing fluency is −.04, p < .01.*

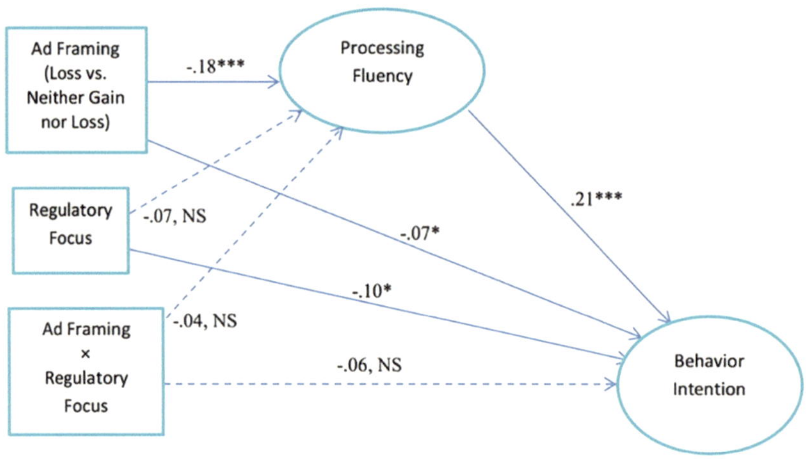

Figure 4.
*Final model (ad framing: Loss vs. neither gain nor loss). Note: 1. χ2 (18) = 32.872, p < .05; CFI = .995; TLI = .991; RMSEA = .027. 2. The model was evaluated by using loss framing as the reference group. 3. * indicates p < .05, ** indicates p < .01, *** indicates p < .001. 4. Dotted line indicates the effect is not statistically significant at 95% level of confidence. 5. The indirect effect of loss vs. neither gain nor loss framing on behavioral intention through processing fluency is −.08, p < .001.*

In addition, processing fluency mediated both the effect of ad framing (gain vs. neutral) and the effect of ad framing (loss vs. neutral) on people's behavioral intention: Processing fluency significantly affected people's behavioral intention, $\beta = .21$, $p < .001$. The indirect effect of ad framing (gain vs. neutral) on behavioral intention through processing fluency was significant ($\gamma = -.03$, $p < .01$). The indirect effect of ad framing (loss vs. neutral) on behavioral intention through processing fluency was also significant ($\gamma = -.08$, $p < .001$).

Based on the results, the statistical diagrams of the final model were presented as follows (See **Figures 2–4**).

5. Discussion

The purpose of this study was to investigate the effectiveness of advertising on people's intentions to control sugar intake. Specifically, three types of ad framing were examined: gain vs. loss vs. neither gain nor loss framing. Moreover, the moderator role of individuals' regulatory focus (promotion focus vs. prevention focus) on the effects of ad framing was explored. In addition, processing fluency was tested as a mediator.

By considering the influences of all tested variables in a whole SEM model, it was found that gain framing was more effective than loss framing in leading people to have greater intentions to limit sugar intake. The positive reaction toward gain-framed ads may be because people do not want to be told not to eat sugar: Many people may find it pleasant to consume sweets and foods with sugar, and limiting sugar intake is a prevention behavior that asks people to give up some kind of pleasure in order to pursue other desirable outcomes. Therefore, using a positive blueprint to persuade them to pursue desirable outcomes may be more effective than using negative illustrations to scare them into giving up their current pleasure.

The findings also showed that both gain and loss framing were more persuasive than the neutral framing in changing peoples' intentions to limit sugar intake. These findings suggest that ad framing (gain vs. loss vs. neither gain nor loss) matters in leading people to have greater intentions to adopt the recommended behavior of limiting sugar intake. Among the three types of ad framing, the neutral framing without emphasizing gain or loss cannot persuade people effectively to reduce sugar intake, while gain framing is the most effective framing to increase people's intention to eat less sugar.

Moreover, there was a significant interaction effect between ad framing (gain vs. loss) and regulatory focus on people's behavioral intentions. Gain framing was more effective in leading promotion-focused individuals to have greater intentions to limit sugar intake than loss framing, while loss framing was more effective in leading prevention-focused individuals to have greater behavioral intentions than gain framing. Based on regulatory focus theory [12], this result may indicate that gain-framed and loss-framed ads separately match people's promotion regulatory focus and prevention focus, which in turn create regulatory fit and lead people to feel right about the message. Therefore, regulatory focus is a moderator in the effects of ad framing (gain vs. loss) on behavioral intention.

Additionally, it was found that processing fluency mediated both the effects of ad framing (gain vs. neutral) and ad framing (loss vs. neutral) on people's behavioral intention to control sugar intake. That is, compared to the neutral-framed ads, both gain- and loss-framed ads were easier for participants to process, and then the greater processing fluency further led to greater advertising persuasiveness. This may be because people already have some knowledge or common sense about the negative consequences of high sugar intake or positive outcomes of controlling sugar intake; thus, compared to the neutral framing, they may process gain and loss framing more fluently with their existing knowledge, and then were better persuaded by the message.

This research provided several implications. The findings insinuate that to persuade the general population (i.e., without knowing their regulatory orientation) to control sugar intake, gain-framed advertising would be the best choice. Instead of always stressing the bad consequences of high sugar consumption to scare people, health professionals should design some positive-framed messages that stress the benefits of lowering sugar intake to stimulate people's stronger desires to control their sugar consumption. Moreover, neutral framing of neither gain nor loss is not a good choice to persuade people to lower their sugar intake. However, if possible, it should be encouraged to find out people's regulatory orientation in order to better persuade them. For example, hospitals or other health organizations can ask obese patients or the patients with high blood sugar to fill out a questionnaire to know their regulatory focus; and then the health professionals can use different strategies tailored to different patients to help them control sugar intake. Specifically, gain-framed messages could be used more often for promotion-focused people, while loss-framed messages should get the priority to be selected for prevention-focused people. In addition, since the findings showed that processing fluency can increase message persuasiveness, making the messages easy to process should be a way to better persuade people to lower sugar intake.

6. Conclusion

Controlling sugar intake is important for individuals since today many people have an appetite disorder [37–39]. The chronical diseases associated with sugar consumption such as obesity and diabetes are epidemic globally [37, 38]. While sugar stimulates individuals' appetites, it also threatens public health if people appetite dysregulation and take excessive sugar [37, 38]. From a communication perspective, the present research contributes to this issue by investigating how to frame advertising messages to more effectively persuade individuals to actively reduce sugar consumptions. Prevention is better cure. More future research could be conducted to help individuals control sugar intake and build better health conditions.

Author details

Kang Li
Zayed University, Abu Dhabi, UAE

*Address all correspondence to: kang.li@zu.ac.ae

References

[1] Johnson, R. K., Appel, L. J., Brands, M., Howard, B. V., Lefevre, M., Lustig, R. H., ... and Wylie-Rosett, J. (2009). Dietary sugars intake and cardiovascular health a scientific statement from the american heart association. Circulation, 120(11), 1011-1020.

[2] Null, G. (2014, March 13). Sugar: killing us sweetly. Staggering health consequences of sugar on health of Americans. Global Research. Retrieved from http://www.globalresearch.ca/sugar-killing-us-sweetly/5367250

[3] Branswell, H. (2014, March 5). Eating sugar causes massive health problems, says WHO. The Canadian Press. Retrieved from http://www.huffingtonpost.ca/2014/03/05/eating-sugar_n_4903790.html

[4] Jung, W. S., & Villegas, J. (2011). The effects of message framing, involvement, and nicotine dependence on anti-smoking public service announcements. Health Marketing Quarterly, 28(3), 219-231.

[5] Covey, J. (2014). The role of dispositional factors in moderating message framing effects. Health Psychology, 33(1), 52-65.

[6] O'Keefe, D. J., & Jensen, J. D. (2006). The advantages of compliance or the disadvantages of noncompliance? A meta-analytic review of the relative persuasive effectiveness of gain-framed and loss-framed messages. Communication Yearbook, 30, 1-43.

[7] O'Keefe, D. J., & Jensen, J. D. (2007). The relative persuasiveness of gain-framed and loss-framed messages for encouraging disease prevention behaviors: A meta-analytic review. Journal of Health Communication, 12(7), 623-644.

[8] O'Keefe, D. J., & Jensen, J. D. (2009). The relative persuasiveness of gain-framed and loss-framed messages for encouraging disease detection behaviors: A meta-analytic review. Journal of Communication, 59, 296-316.

[9] O'Keefe, D. J., & Jensen, J. D. (2010). The relative effectiveness of gain-framed and loss-framed persuasive appeals concerning obesity related behaviors: Meta-analytic evidence and implications. In R. Batra, P. A. Keller, & V. J. Strecher (Eds.), Leveraging consumer psychology for effective health communications (pp. 171-185). Armonk, NY: M. E. Sharpe Inc.

[10] Gallagher, K. M., & Updegraff, J. A. (2012). Health message framing effects on attitudes, intentions, and behavior: A meta-analytic review. Annals of Behavioral Medicine, 43(1), 101-116.

[11] Latimer, A. E., Salovey, P., & Rothman, A. J. (2007). The effectiveness of gain-framed messages for encouraging disease prevention behavior: Is all hope lost? Journal of Health Communication, 12(7), 645-649.

[12] Higgins, E. T. (1997). Beyond pleasure and pain. American Psychologist, 52(12), 1280-1300.

[13] Higgins, E. T. (1999). Promotion and prevention as a motivational duality: Implications for evaluative processes. In S. Chaiken and Y. Trope (Eds.), Dual-process theories in social psychology (pp. 503-525). New York, NY: The Guilford Press.

[14] Lee, A. Y., and Aaker, J. L. (2004). Bringing the frame into focus: The influence of regulatory fit on processing fluency and persuasion. Journal of Personality and Social Psychology, 86(2), 205-218.

[15] Zhao, G., & Pechmann, C. (2007). The impact of regulatory focus on adolescents' response to antismoking

advertising campaigns. Journal of Marketing Research, 44(4), 671-687.

[16] Vaughn, L. A., Childs, K. E., Maschinski, C., Niño, N. P., and Ellsworth, R. (2010). Regulatory fit, processing fluency, and narrative persuasion. Social and Personality Psychology Compass, 4(12), 1181-1192.

[17] Rothman, A. J., Bartels, R. D., Wlaschin, J., & Salovey, P. (2006). The strategic use of gain- and loss-framed messages to promote healthy behavior: How theory can inform practice. Journal of Communication, 56, S202-S220.

[18] Meyerowitz, B. E., & Chaiken, S. (1987). The effect of message framing on breast self-examination attitudes, intentions, and behavior. Journal of Personality and Social Psychology, 52(3), 500-510.

[19] Rothman, A. J., Salovey, P., Antone, C., Keough, K., & Martin, C. D. (1993). The influence of message framing on intentions to perform health behaviors. Journal of Experimental Social Psychology, 29(5), 408-433.

[20] Banks, S. M., Salovey, P., Greener, S., Rothman, A. J., Moyer, A., Beauvais, J., & Epel, E. (1995). The effects of message framing on mammography utilization. Health Psychology, 14(2), 178-184.

[21] Millar, M. G., & Millar, K. U. (2000). Promoting safe driving behaviors: The influences of message framing and issue involvement. Journal of Applied Social Psychology, 30(4), 853-866.

[22] Cox, D., & Cox, A. D. (2001). Communicating the consequences of early detection: The role of evidence and framing. Journal of Marketing, 65(3), 91-103.

[23] Schneider, T. R., Salovey, P., Apanovitch, A. M., Pizarro, J., McCarthy, D., Zullo, J., & Rothman, A. J. (2001). The effects of message framing and ethnic targeting on mammography use among low-income women. Health Psychology, 20(4), 256-266.

[24] Finney, L. J., & Iannotti, R. J. (2002). Message framing and mammography screening: A theory-driven intervention. Behavioral Medicine, 28(1), 5-14.

[25] Higgins, E. T. (2002). How self-regulation creates distinct values: The case of promotion and prevention decision making. Journal of Consumer Psychology, 12(3), 177-191.

[26] Cesario, J., Higgins, E. T., and Scholer, A. A. (2008). Regulatory fit and persuasion: Basic principles and remaining questions. Social and Personality Psychology Compass, 2(1), 444-463.

[27] Higgins, E. T. (2000). Making a good decision: Value from fit. American Psychologist, 55(11), 1217-1230.

[28] Cesario, J., Grant, H., & Higgins, E. T. (2004). Regulatory fit and persuasion: Transfer from 'feeling right'. Journal of Personality and Social Psychology, 86(3), 388-404.

[29] Grewal, D., Motyka, S., Puccinelli, N. M., Roggeveen, A. L., Daryanto, A., de Ruyter, K., and Wetzels, M. (2011). Understanding how to achieve competitive advantage through regulatory fit: a meta-analysis. Marketing Science Institute Research Report, 10-117.

[30] Uskul, A. K., Sherman, D. K., & Fitzgibbon, J. (2009). The cultural congruency effect: Culture, regulatory focus, and the effectiveness of gain- vs. loss-framed health messages. Journal of Experimental Social Psychology,45(3), 535-541.

[31] Lee, A. Y. (2001). The mere exposure effect: An uncertainty reduction explanation revisited. Personality and Social Psychology Bulletin, 27(10), 1255-1266.

[32] Whittlesea, B. W. A. (1993). Illusions of familiarity. Journal of Experimental Psychology: Learning, Memory, and Cognition, 19(6), 1235-1253.

[33] Reber, R., Winkielman, P., & Schwarz, N. (1998). Effects of perceptual fluency on affective judgments. Psychological Science, 9(1), 45-48.

[34] Lee, A. Y., Keller, P. A., and Sternthal, B. (2010). Value from regulatory construal fit: The persuasive impact of fit between consumer goals and message concreteness. Journal of Consumer Research, 36(5), 735-747.

[35] Labroo, A. A., and Lee, A. Y. (2006). Between two brands: A goal fluency account of brand evaluation. Journal of Marketing Research, 43(3), 374-385.

[36] Muthén, L., and Muthén, B. (2012). MPLUS (7). Los Angeles, CA: Muthén and Muthén.

[37] Martins, I. J. (2013). Appetite dysregulation and obesity in Western Countries: Food restriction maintains the health and well-being of overweight individuals. Germany: LAP Lambert Academic Publishing.

[38] Martins, I. J. (2020). Appetite dysregulation and the apelinergic system are connected to global chronic disease epidemic. Series of Endocrinology, Diabetes and Metabolism. 1(3), 67-69.

[39] Martins, I. J. (2015). Nutritional diets accelerate amyloid beta metabolism and prevent the induction of chronic diseases and Alzheimer's disease. Photon ebooks.

Chapter 7

Fructose Intake: Metabolism and Role in Diseases

Luke He, Ghufran S. Babar, Jacob M. Redel, Sabetha L. Young, Callie E. Chagas, Wayne V. Moore and Yun Yan

Abstract

Fructose consumption has dramatically increased worldwide over the past decades. There are numerous clinical, experimental, and epidemiological studies evidenced that increased consumption of fructose negatively impacts carbohydrate metabolism and lactate formed from fructose can also affect whole-body energy balance. Excessive fructose intake stimulates endogenous glucose production and lipid synthesis in the liver. Currently fructose is believed to be a major contributing factor to chronic metabolic diseases, including obesity, insulin resistance, hypertriglyceridemia, and non-alcoholic fatty liver disease, hyperglycemia, type 2 diabetes, and cancer. These new findings bring challenges to researchers today because of what is still to be discovered, and how to apply what has been discovered to modern health. Further investigation should seek to analyze and understand specific mechanistic effects of fructose in metabolic pathways, and how to apply this knowledge to our daily lives. Conducting this monosaccharide research is important to improve the diet of the general population and to attenuate the epidemics of metabolic disease and associated diseases. Here, we focus on the mechanism and role of fructose in diseases as well as its potential as a dietary interventional target.

Keywords: fructose, glucose, sucrose, obesity, insulin resistance, uric acid, hypertriglyceridemia, hyperglycemia, type 2 diabetes, hypertension, retinopathy, free oxygen radicals, cancer

1. Introduction

Fructose is a common form of sugar found naturally in fruits, honey, and table sugar. It is often used as an additive to modern foods and drinks. Its sweetening effects and low costs of production have made fructose increasingly popular [1, 2]. Fructose consumption has increased since the 1970s. Mean fructose intake per person increased approximately 32% from the 1970s to early 2000s. Of note, total carbohydrate intake over that period increased by 41%, indicating an increase in glucose consumption as well [3]. In a 2008 study analyzing fructose consumption of 21,483 people, the mean fructose intake per capita was about 54.7 g/day (10.2% of total caloric intake/day) [1]. Dietary Guidelines for Americans 2015–2020 recommended that average intake of added sugars should be less than 10% of total calories per day [4]. Worldwide the consumption of sugar varies by age, setting and county. Among different European countries, for example, intake ranges widely, from 7 to 25% of total energy intake [5].

Fructose intake in the diet has been linked to certain human diseases [6–10]. However, the precise role of fructose in disease is poorly understood and some findings are still controversial. There are numerous studies associating fructose with negative impacts on multiple components of metabolism in animals and humans [11–14]. The past few decades of research have expanded our understanding of fructose, yet there is still much to learn. It is important to establish an accurate scientific understanding of fructose and its implications on human health because of its increasing popularity worldwide. This chapter focuses on up to date findings related to the metabolism and the role of fructose in human disease, including hypertension, hyperglycemia, metabolic syndrome, free oxygen radicals, retinopathy, diabetes, and cancer.

2. Structure, uses, and metabolism

Fructose is one of three major monosaccharides consumed by humans, in addition to glucose and galactose. Its catabolism produces the same energy content as glucose, 4 kilocalories per gram. Fructose is found as a monosaccharide in honey and fruits. It is found as part of the disaccharide sucrose in cane sugar, used to make table sugar. Sucrose is comprised of glucose bound to fructose in a 1:1 ratio (**Figure 1**). Fructose, a potent sweetener, is also artificially added to foods and sugar-sweetened beverages (SSB), often in the form of high fructose corn syrup (HFCS). HFCS refers to the fructose content relative to corn syrup, which is entirely glucose, rather than the fructose content relative to other sweeteners. Indeed, as in sucrose and in honey, most HFCS compounds used as food additives contain nearly the same 1:1 ratio of glucose to fructose. Therefore, it is important to understand that concerns pertaining to fructose consumption might also be inferred to a wide range of sweeteners, not only HFCS.

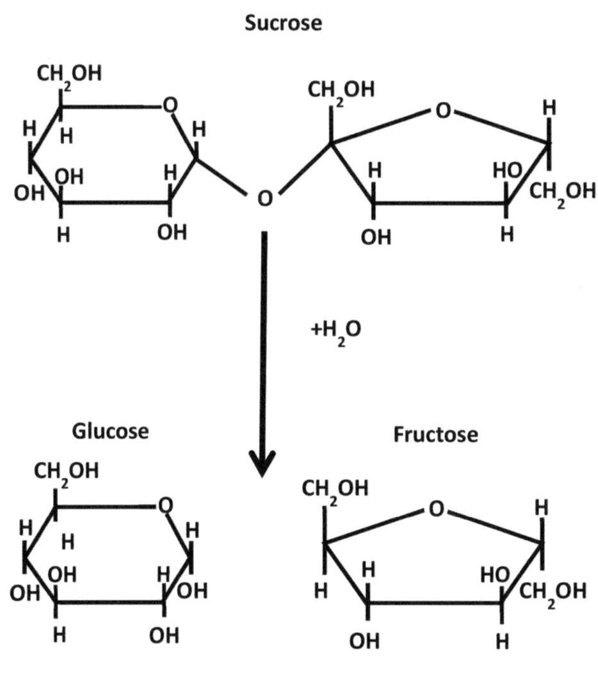

Figure 1.
Structural formula of the sucrose, glucose and fructose. Sucrose is a disaccharide consisting of one glucose and one fructose molecule. Hydrolysis breaks the glycoside bond converting sucrose into glucose and fructose.

Digestive and intestinal brush border enzymes break down polysaccharides and disaccharides into monosaccharides—fructose, glucose, or galactose. Free fructose is absorbed directly from the intestinal lumen and is transported into circulation primarily by glucose transporter 5 (GLUT5) and glucose transporter 2 (GLUT2). Once in the portal circulation, almost all absorbed fructose enters the liver [15]. Fructose is transported into hepatocytes primarily via hepatic GLUT2. In addition, other family members of glucose transporters are involved in fructose absorption and metabolism [16]. After ingestion into liver, fructose is metabolized to either glucose [17], glyceraldehyde or acetyl CoA [18]. The liver distributes energy to other cells in the form of glucose, lactate, and triglycerides or converts this energy into hepatic glycogen or fat (**Figure 2**) [19, 20].

Extrahepatic fructose metabolism is generally considered minimal. Extrahepatic cells do not express fructokinase, so fructose metabolism must be catalyzed by hexokinase in these cells. Hexokinase has a much higher affinity for glucose than fructose. Thus, conversion from fructose to fructose 6-phosphate proceeds slowly in extrahepatic cells, preventing them from playing a large role in fructose metabolism [21].

Under diabetic conditions, excess glucose may enter the polyol pathway and can be converted to exogenous fructose (**Figure 3**). In this pathway, aldose reductase reduces glucose to sorbitol and NADPH is oxidized to $NADP^+$. Sorbitol dehydrogenase then oxidizes sorbitol to fructose, which produces NADH from NAD^+ [6, 22, 23]. The polyol pathway can result in NADH/NAD^+ redox imbalances in diabetes [22]. Excessive activation of this pathway increases reactive oxygen species (ROS), and decreases nitric oxide (NO) and glutathione, promoting microvascular damage to the retina, kidney and nerves [24–27].

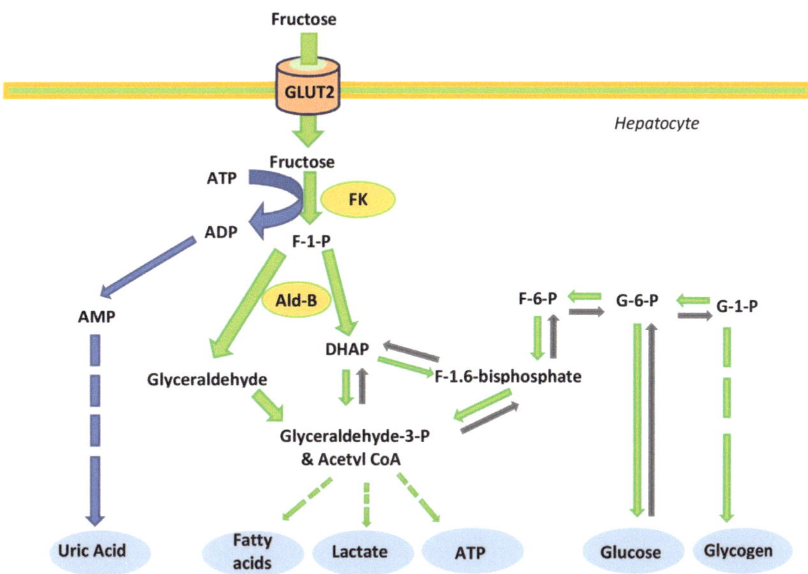

Figure 2.
Fructose metabolism in hepatocyte: After absorption from intestine, fructose is taken by hepatocyte via the glucose transporter 2 (GLUT2) and rapidly converted to fructose-1-phosphate (F-1-P) by fructokinase. F-1-P is then metabolized to glyceraldehyde or dihydroxyacetone phosphate (DHAP) via aldolase B (Ald-B). Glyceraldehyde will be further converted to glyceraldehyde-3-phosphate and acetyle CoA, finally will convert to fat acids, lactate or ATP. In liver, F-1-P also can convert into glucose and glycogen via DHAP and glyceraldehyde-3-p to improve glycogenesis. In addition, intracellular phosphate levels decrease stimulates formation of uric acid and increases the level of uric acid at blood. F-6-P; fructose-6 phosphate, G-6-P; glucose-6-phosphate; G-1-P, glucose-1-phosphate.

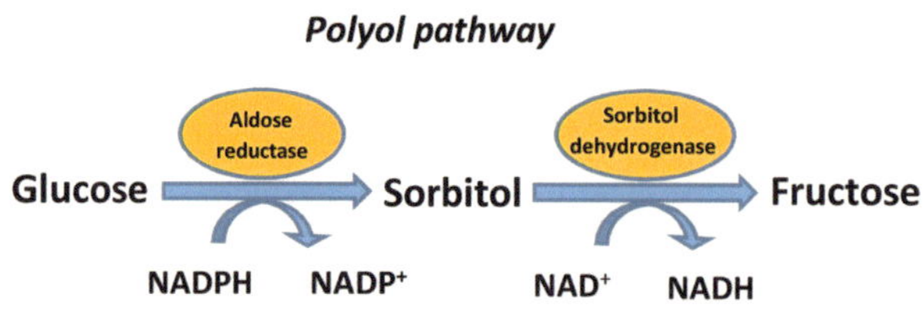

Figure 3.
Polyol pathway: Under normal physiological conditions, glucose is used for energy (ATP) production via glycolysis. In diabetes, excess glucose enters the polyol pathway. Aldose reductase reduces glucose to sorbital and oxidizes NADPH to $NADP^+$, then sorbitol dehydrogenase oxidizes sorbitol to fructose, which produces NADH from NAD^+.

3. Free oxygen radicals and endothelial dysfunction

By comparing the aorta of rats exposed to fructose with controls exposed to mannitol and testing them with the superoxide anion scavenger superoxide dismutase (SOD), fructose has the effect of inducing NADPH-derived superoxide anion production. SOD incubation increased the response to acetylcholine in the fructose-exposed group. The group exposed to fructose showed a leftward shift in the concentration-response curve to acetylcholine when apocynin was added, but the group exposed to mannitol did not. Additionally, the concentration response curves for both groups to phenylephrine were shifted to the right after SOD incubation, but this effect was greater in the fructose-exposed group [28]. In addition, it was found that high-fructose diet (HFrD) increased ROS 2.8 times in the aorta of rat [29]. Another study found that fructose increased blood pressure, superoxide anion, and expression of NADPH oxidase subunits $p47^{phox}$ and $p22^{phox}$ in rat endothelium [30].

Fructose can induce expression of the pro-inflammatory molecule intracellular adhesion molecule-1 (ICAM-1) on human and rat endothelial cells. This is due to a fructose-induced reduction of endothelial NO synthase (eNOS) expression [31]. Moreover, eNOS gene therapy helped repress the damaging the effect induced by a HFrD, indicating that eNOS has a protective effect [32]. HFrD can impair cardiac AKT/eNOS signaling. In contrast, estradiol can activate the Akt/eNOS signaling that is impaired by HFrD in rat heart [33].

The effect of topical fructose and dextrose on the adherence of leukocyte adherence in rat mesenteric venules was observed with intravital microscopy. The result showed that fructose induced significant inflammation, but dextrose did not. It was determined that fructose was mediating endothelial damage via ROS generation because the damage was blocked by NO donors spermine NONO-ate and antioxidant lipoic acid [34]. A recent study in human endothelial cells found that exposure to high fructose concentrations significantly affected gene expression, decreased the cellular angiogenic capability, and impaired endothelial vascular function [35].

4. Hypertension

Several articles have reviewed the effects of fructose on blood pressure (BP) [36, 37]. Various mechanisms have been proposed, including increased sympathetic activation [38], inflammation [31], endothelial dysfunction [39], increased uric acid stimulation [40], inhibition of eNOS system [32], increased salt and water retention [41, 42], increased homocysteine levels [43] and in utero programmed hypertension of offspring [44].

Few epidemiological studies have examined the association between fructose intake, uric acid, and BP levels. Some studies have conflicting conclusions about the relationship between fructose and blood pressure [45]. A cross-sectional epidemiological study using the data collected from the National Health and Nutrition Examination Survey indicated that a high intake of fructose of ≥74 g/day is associated with elevated BP in the adults without a medical history of hypertension [39]. Studies have shown that HFrD of 60% fructose chow in rats leads to hypertension [46]. Recent epidemiological studies [39, 45] and meta-analysis [47] have indicated that there is an association between fructose and BP. In addition, when fructose is provided in a beverage, there is an acute BP raising effect [37, 48]. Moreover, lowering sugar-sweetened beverages intake was significantly associated with reduced BP in adults with hypertension [49]. There may also be epigenetic impact, because the HFrD of pregnant women was associated with BP programming in the offspring [44, 50].

In a mouse model, high salt intake caused leptin resistance and obesity by stimulating endogenous fructose production and metabolism. It also raised BP and induced metabolic syndrome which was abrogated when fructose metabolism was blocked [51]. It was found that after 30 minutes of 40 mM fructose exposure on the rat aorta, with and without the endothelium lining, the contractile responses induced by phenylephrine (a selective α_1–adrenergic receptor agonist) were increased in the rat aorta with endothelium present. This demonstrated that the effects of fructose on contractile response resulted from fructose acting on the endothelium and not the smooth muscle [28]. NO, an important vasodilator, was shown to have reduced availability when NO synthase was blocked with L-NAME. The result showed that a smaller shift occurred in NO production in the aorta segments exposed to fructose ranging from 0 to 40 mM concentrations. It was also shown that fructose increased activation of NADPH oxidase of the aorta, leading to production of superoxide anions and less NO bioavailability. The NO bioavailability may also be affected by hydrogen peroxide, which is known as an endogenous regulator of NO synthase [52]. Catalase, a hydrogen peroxide scavenger, was used to study the rat aorta segments. The results showed that catalase reduced the vasodilatory response to acetylcholine only in the rings incubated with mannitol, and not with fructose. This suggests that the vasodilator effects of hydrogen peroxide were impaired after fructose exposure. Additionally, catalase reduced the response to phenylephrine in the aorta incubated with fructose, suggesting that fructose increased hydrogen peroxide, leading to increased contractility [28]. Fructose may also reduce NO bioavailability by generating uric acid, which reduces NO levels by blocking L-arginine uptake, stimulating arginase, inhibiting eNOS, and by direct scavenging [53, 54]. Fructose can enhance expression of apical chloride/base exchanger Slc26a6 (PAT1, CFEX), which increased salt and water absorption, Slc26a6 and Glut5 play an essential role in fructose-inducing hypertension [41].

The National Health and Nutrition Examination Survey (NHANEX 2003 to 2006) examined the relationship between increased fructose intake and blood pressure in healthy adults. Their study consisted of 2253 diverse participants and showed that a high fructose intake (defined as >74 g/day) was associated with elevated blood pressure levels, both with and without adjusting for numerous risk factors. The results showed 26%, 30%, and 77% higher risk for the blood pressure cut offs: ≥135/85, ≥140/90, and ≥ 160/100 mmHg, respectively [39].

5. Dyslipidemia and obesity

The conversion of fructose to fat in the liver (de novo lipogenesis) may be a modifiable pathogenic pathway [55]. Fructose uptake increases triglycerides by conversion to trioses-phosphate. Tests in rats [43, 46] and humans [18, 56] have shown that HFrD increase triglycerides. HFrD also increases fasting plasma triglycerides level and the diet significantly inhibited several pathways of lipid metabolism [57]. It increased plasma triglycerides in both males and females, but with a higher degree in males [58]. In obese individuals it increased triglycerides more than glucose [18].

In a rat animal model, HFrD for 5 weeks significantly increased plasma triglycerides (3.8-fold) and decreased high-density lipoprotein cholesterol by 14% [59]. Consuming fructose-sweetened beverages for 10 weeks has shown a significant increase in visceral adipose tissue, dyslipidemia, and an impaired glucose tolerance compared to the corresponding glucose cohorts, although weight gain was not different in either cohorts [60, 61].

The prevalence of overweight status and obesity in children has increased dramatically in recent decades. SSB is already a known risk factor for weight gain in children and adults [62, 63]. Numerous prospective cohort studies have illustrated that increasing intake of SSB contributes to obesity [62, 64–66], while reducing the intake of soft drinks can reduce weight [67]. HFrD promoted metabolic syndrome by inducing lipogenesis and causing triglyceride accumulation and insulin resistance [68]. Oxidative stress and inflammation due to HFrD also induced metabolic changes [6, 68]. Hyperhomocysteinemia is also associated with the changes seen in the individuals with metabolic syndrome [69]. Rats fed with high fructose for 5 weeks had 72% higher homocysteine levels compared to chow fed controls. Rats fed with HFrD developed metabolic syndrome, which includes hypertriglyceridemia and obesity [43].

6. Non-alcoholic fatty liver disease

The liver is essential for metabolism of proteins, fats, and carbohydrates. Liver disease may affect various components of metabolism and may contribute to metabolic syndrome. Non-alcoholic fatty liver disease (NAFLD) or non-alcoholic steatohepatitis (NASH) can result from excessive fat accumulation in the liver leading to liver damage and inflammation. NAFLD is a manifestation of metabolic syndrome. NAFLD affects about 30–40% of the adult population [70] and about 10% children [71]. Persistent liver damage can cause cirrhosis and hepatocellular carcinoma [72].

An imbalance in fatty acid synthesis, β-oxidation, and triglyceride exportation processes leads to the accumulation of fat in hepatocytes. Fructose is a substrate and inducer of hepatic de novo lipogenesis [6]. Fructose has a role in inducing fatty liver disease by stimulating carbohydrates conversion into fatty acids and blocking β-fatty acid oxidation [73]. As mentioned previously, fructose is converted into glyceraldehyde-3-phosphate by avoiding the rate-controlling step of glucose metabolism in hepatocytes. Thus, the consumption of high fructose increases the hepatic de novo lipogenesis [74]. Excessive lipogenesis causes hepatic inflammation, a key pathophysiologic feature of NASH [75]. These processes also increase mitochondrial coupling, leading to oxidative stress [74]. Numerous studies have shown that fructose uptake causes ATP depletion because it floods the hepatocytes with fructose-1-phosphate via fructokinase [76–78].

The effects of fructose consumption on NAFLD and metabolic syndrome have been studied [79, 80]. Increased fructose consumption has been suggested to contribute to NAFLD [81, 82]. A study on zebra fish showed that when treated with 4% fructose or glucose, only the fructose-treated larvae developed NASH [83].

Fructose intake also affects insulin sensitivity and has been shown to increase fibrosis severity in patients who have NASH [84]. Short term (9 days) high fructose intake of 25% of energy content was associated with increased hepatic fatty acid synthesis and liver fat in healthy men fed weight-maintaining diets [85]. There have been retrospective studies done on patients with NAFLD, showing that they correlate with a higher fructose intake, despite similar overall energy intake compared to healthy individuals. Another meta-analysis concluded that consumption of SSB plays a role in fatty liver disease [67]. However, results are not conclusive. A recent meta-analysis of six observational and 21 intervention studies concluded that the apparent association between indices of human health like liver fat and lipogenesis from fructose or sucrose intake appear to be confounded by excessive energy intake overall [86].

Increasing evidences show that Sirtuin 1 (Sirt1) plays a vital role in the development and rescue of NAFLD [87]. Sirt1 is a NAD^+-dependent histone deacetylase and is considered to be a core regulator in fatty acid oxidation and lipogenesis [88, 89]. Sirt1 reduces liver steatosis, improves mitochondrial function, and restores insulin sensitivity, thereby improving blood sugar and lipid regulation [90]. In addition, Sirt1 has anti-inflammatory activity, anti-aging activity and reduces oxidative stress of the vascular endothelium. Enhancing Sirt1 activation can reduce lipogenic enzymes expression [91] and lipid accumulation in liver [92]. Ablating the Skirt1 activation can exacerbate liver fat accumulation and hepatic steatosis [93, 94]. Diet has been shown to be involved in the regulation of Sirt1. An unhealthy diet can increase the risk of NAFLD and obesity [93, 94]. Nutritional and lifestyle interventions can increase the activation of Sirt1 and improve NAFLD [94, 95]. Fructose decreases the expression and activity of Sirt1 in liver, and inhibits lipid metabolism [96], whereas increased Sirt1 activity can attenuate fructose-induced hepatic lipid deposition and prevent NAFLD [90]. In high-fat diet mice, activation of the AMPK/Sirt1 pathway significantly improved obesity, lipid accumulation and hepatic steatosis [97]. In addition, metformin has been proposed to alleviate NAFLD, since metformin can increase autophagy by increasing the expression and activation of the Sirt1 [92].

In recent years, Sirt1 activators and inhibitors have been extensively studied, including some human trails [98, 99]. Ongoing research data suggests that NAFLD may benefit from targeting Sirt1 therapy [98].

7. Insulin resistance

Fructose consumption can result in insulin resistance, an effect that is similar to glucose [13]. In rats, high fructose consumption resulted in increased visceral adipose tissue, insulin resistance and hypertension [100, 101]. A higher C-peptide is often associated with insulin resistance [102]. A study was conducted to evaluate the link between fructose intake and C-peptide level in women, and it found that the serum C-peptide concentration of the subjects with the highest intake of fructose was 13.9% higher than those with the lowest intake [103]. In rats fed with HFrD resulted in a complete metabolic syndrome including hyperinsulinemia [43].

Fructose also sensitized pancreatic beta cells to TNF-alpha induced necroptosis [104]. Fructose showed increased insulin resistance in both obese men and women, more notable in males [58]. Fructose increased visceral adipose tissue, plasma insulin, blood triglyceride level, and HOMA index. There was a decreased stimulation of protein kinase B signaling in fructose fed rats. Insulin induced GLUT4 presence on plasma membranes of cardiac cells was decreased by fructose diet [105].

The body's use of insulin may be impaired by increased resistance in peripheral tissues, it is important to assess the effects of fructose on the insulin and the pancreatic beta cells. It is well known that hyperglycemia is detrimental to beta-cell viability, which is a large part of the pathophysiology of development for diabetes mellitus. One factor in the beta cell death is a mitochondrial channel called the permeability transition pore (PTP, or MTP). PTP is associated with mitochondrial dysfunction and directly involved in insulin resistance [106]. There is evidence that PTP inhibitors prevent the pancreatic β cell death induced by hyperglycemia [107]. Comparing the effects of fructose and glucose on PTP, the results show that even low concentration of fructose (2.5 mM) can induce PTP open, similar to 30 mM glucose [108]. This indicated that the possible role of fructose on PTP and in the development of beta cell damage.

8. Diabetes

In healthy people, acute increases in plasma glucose concentration inhibit endogenous glucose production. This regulation is disrupted in type 2 diabetes patients, causing inappropriate endogenous glucose production and hyperglycemia [109]. Hyperglycemia inhibits glucose production when an intracellular influx of glucose is catalyzed to glucose-6-phosphate via glucokinase [110]. In healthy individuals, there is an autoregulatory mechanism in which glucose phosphorylation suppresses glucose production, primarily by inhibiting glycogenolysis [111].

Studies show that fructose may have an impact on glucose level. In one study, dogs were fasted for 42 hours, then they were administered different amounts of IV fructose. Fructose exposure caused an increase in net hepatic glucose uptake, glycogen synthesis and hepatic lactate output, the experiments show that about 70% of H3- labeled glucose captured by the liver is incorporated into glycogen and deposited in liver [112]. This is significant because glucokinase is known to activate the glycogen synthase enzyme [113]. Fructose has a role in determining glucokinase activity, glucokinase has a major role in determining hepatic glucose uptake [112].

Other animal studies have shown that after two weeks of high fructose intake, blood glucose levels were significantly increased in healthy rats [114]. A study in humans has shown small amounts of fructose stimulated hepatic glucose uptake and hepatic glycogen synthesis. Under euglycemic hyperinsulinemia, low-dose fructose infusion increased net hepatic glycogen synthesis by 3 times via stimulating glycogen synthase flux [115]. Glucose-fructose co-ingestion will significantly increase hepatic glycogen repletion rates compared with glucose ingestion alone [116].

It is important to understand that although insulin resistance and pancreatic cell damage may develop in rats fed with HFrD as reported by some studies, the presentations might not always mimic type 2 diabetes found in humans or rats. For example, HFrD combined with high fat diet to induce T2D in rodents. These animals only developed early stage of diabetes but did not develop β-cell failure as seen in the late stages of T2D in humans [117, 118]. The animal could develop a nutritional tolerance after eating a fructose diet for 3 months, but these animals could be not used as suitable fructose-fed animal model for diabetes study due to no signs of insulin resistance and β-cell dysfunction [119]. A new and alternative rat model was created by using a 10% fructose-fed diet followed by 40 mg/kg of streptozotocin to induce beta cell toxicity. In this animal model, rats developed both insulin resistance and pancreatic β-cell dysfunction [120].

In humans, the epidemic of T2D and diabetes-related metabolic complications have been linked to fructose consumption [121–125]. Indeed, fructose as a highly lipogeneic monosaccharide, fructose intake increases the risk of impairing gluocse metabolism [63, 126]. However, results are conflicting. An excessive rate of endogenous glucose production is a major contributor to fasting hyperglycemia in diabetes. A study on human showed that infusion of small amounts of fructose during hyperglycemia partially corrected the regulation of glucose production and partially restored the ability of glucose to suppress glucose production in subjects with type 2 diabetes [127].

In diabetes mellitus, hyperglycemic condition increases the activity of polyol pathway; approximately 30% glucose can be converted to fructose via the polyol pathway. Persistent hyperglycemia increases fructose level and decreases NADPD/NADP$^+$ ratio, leading to NO production decrease, ROS production increase, oxidative stress, and protein glycation increase. These events damage the microvascular system and are implicated in diabetic complications, especially in retinopathy, nephropathy, and neuropathy [22].

9. Hyperuricemia

Hyperuricemia (HP) can cause metabolic, cardiovascular, and renal diseases [68]. Elevated level of uric acid can inhibit NO bioavailability; it also can promote smooth muscle cell proliferation and can activate the inflammation cascade, which can lead to damage of the endothelium of vessels [128, 129]. During fructose metabolism intracellular phosphate (PO4) is decreased, there is an activation of adenosine monophosphate deaminase which increases inosine monophosphate. Inosine monophosphate is further degraded to xanthine and hypoxanthine by xanthine oxidase (XO). The end product of these processes is uric acid [130, 131] (**Figure 4**). Furthermore, the increased insulin levels due to fructose intake lead to renal reuptake of urate, resulting in reducing the excretion of uric acid through the kidneys and further increases the serum uric acid level [53, 132].

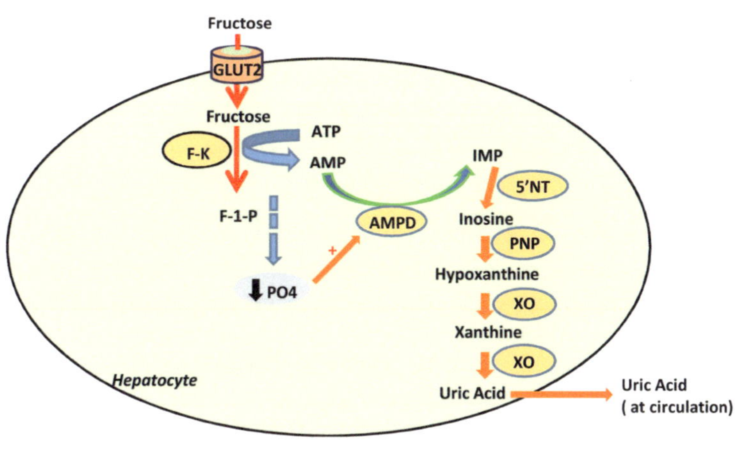

Figure 4.
Fructose stimulates hepatic uric acid synthesis. Fructose is transported into liver via hepatic GLUT2 and is phosphorylated by fructokinase (F-K) to fructose-1-phosphate (F-1-P), which uses ATP as a phosphate donor and results in intracellular phosphate (PO4) depletion. Intracellular phosphate levels decrease stimulates the activity of hepatic AMP deaminase (AMPD). AMPD catalyzes AMP to inosine monophosphate (IMP). IMP is converted to inosine by 5′ nucleotidase (5′NT) and then inosine is further degraded to hypoxanthine by purine nucleotide phosphorylase (PNP). Hypoxanthine is degraded into xanthine by xanthine oxidase (XO), and finally produced uric acid is released into circulation.

A meta-analysis of animal research showed that there is a significant relationship between fructose feeding and HP [133]. Research has also shown that when rats fed with HFrD, elevated uric acid blocked acetylcholine-mediated arterial dilation [53]. Human can also develop HP after high fructose consumption [11, 40, 129]. SSB consumption was significantly associated with increased uric acid concentration in adult population [134]. However, a meta-analysis showed that uric acid concentration was reduced by using glucose instead of fructose [135].

10. Retinopathy

Chronic uncontrolled hyperglycemia can cause microvascular damage which can manifest as diabetic retinopathy (DR). Pathological retinal findings include microaneurysms, capillary abnormalities, hyperpermeability, hypoperfusion, and neo-angiogenesis, which eventually can lead to loss of vision [136, 137].

Animal studies have showed that animals can develop metabolic syndrome while on fructose diet and can also develop choroidal neovascularization which can lead to exudative age-related macular degeneration [137–139]. The retinal neovascularization occurs as part of oxidative stress resulting in an activation and infiltration of phagocytic cells in the retina. High fructose diet can also modulate gene expression in the retina [138]. The genes are involved in the development of diabetic retinopathy [140]. Melatonin plays an important role in the maintenance of disc shedding, function of rod photoreceptors [141], and elongation of cone photoreceptors in the retina [142]. Melatonin also blocks apoptosis of retinal cells after experimentally induced ischemia [143]. Excessive fructose consumption leads to down regulation of melatonin, and decrease the effects of melatonin on anti-inflammation and anti-oxidative stress in the retina [144, 145].

The premature death of retinal pericytes is a pathophysiological hallmark of DR. One study showed that advanced glycosylated end-products (AGEs) can cause retinal pericytes dysfunction and death by reducing survival signals mediated by platelet-derived growth factor [146]. DR is also caused oxidative stress because of increased ROS production and antioxidant depletion [147]. Protein kinase C (PKC) also has an important role in diabetic retinopathy, PKC activation leads to upregulation of pro-inflammatory genes, loss of capillary pericytes and generation of ROS [148, 149].

11. Cancer

Research studies have provided clinical and experimental evidence that fructose intake is associated with development of cancer, especially if consumed in large amounts [150]. Adenomatous polyposis coli (APC) genes can develop biallelic mutations and in combination with fructose intake can trigger or promote the colorectal cancer [151, 152]. The fructose transporter GLUT5 receptors are expressed on the cancer cells like colorectal and breast cancers indicated that fructose can be used as fuel by several types of cancers [153, 154]. Excessive intake of fructose can lead to increased formation of RDS production via formation of glycolaldehyde [155]. Glyoxal is an autoxidation product during fructose metabolism and also a contaminant in the food processing promoted intestinal tumor growth in mouse model.

Fructose was shown to be carcinogenic even if it was only 3% of total daily caloric intake which are mediated through activation of GLUT5 and phosphofructokinase. If fructokinase (ketohexokinase) which is the first enzyme involved in fructose is knocked out in mice the cancer growth can be suppressed [156, 157].

Fructose can also promote cancer growth via pentose phosphate and increases protein synthesis and also cause hepatic inflammation, nonalcoholic fatty liver disease and hepatocellular carcinoma [158, 159].

Fructose promotes cancer growth by formation of lactate, which is an end-product of fructose metabolism. Lactate is likely needed at several steps during the cancer growth including escape from the immune system, cell migration, metastasis and self-sustenance [160]. Lactate levels were found to be 40-fold high in glycolytic tumors and it correlates with cancer cell metastasis and poor survival [161]. Lactate also promotes angiogenesis in the tumors by inducing vascular endothelial growth factor (VEGF) in endothelial cells. If the lactate production is blocked by a chemical inhibitor or gene deletion, the angiogenesis and cancer cell proliferation is stopped [162, 163].

Fructose and uric acid have been shown to stimulate mitochondrial ROS production which is needed for tumor cell growth [164, 165]. During the rapid cell division cancer cells can suffer from hypoxic conditions and have to tolerate them to maintain viability and growth [166]. Fructose metabolism is useful in rapidly dividing cancer cells since during the glycolytic pathway it can use one molecule of ATP to generate 4 molecules of ATP from fructose-1,6-bisphosphate through pyruvate [167].

Fructose consumption may promote breast cancer cell line MDA-MB-468 to an aggressive type [168]. Fructose intake is associated with more aggressive cancer behavior and may promote metastasis [168–170]. Fructose also has a role in pancreatic cancer growth via the induction of transketolase flux [171]. Prostate cancer cell may also use fructose as the preferred energy source to support the cell proliferation and metabolism [172].

Human cells have the ability to produce fructose endogenously, which is also possible in the cancer cells [173]. Endogenous fructose production takes place through the polyol pathway by utilizing aldolase reductase. This enzyme is found in an activated state in various types of human cancers, including liver, breast, ovarian, cervical, and rectal cancers and helps in synthesizing fructose from glucose [174].

Fructose can promote cancer cell growth by providing fuel to make nucleotides, lipids, and energy, especially for cancers that express GLUT5 receptors. Low fructose diet and fructokinase inhibitors can be novel techniques to treat cancers. Furthermore, blocking uric acid and lactate production could also be targets of cancer prevention and treatment [175].

12. Summary

The past decade of research on fructose has expanded our understanding of role of fructose in disease. The imbalance between high fructose intake and low physical energy consumption is a possible reason of the deleterious health effect of fructose. The consumption of excess fructose may promote the development of metabolic disorders directly or indirectly. Dietary fructose intake has been linked with some human diseases, including hypertension, obesity, dyslipidemia, diabetes, non-alcoholic fatty liver syndrome, and certain type of cancers. Further investigation to gain a better understanding about fructose metabolism will be important to define a potential dietary intervention to reduce disease.

Conflict of interest

The authors declare that there is no conflict of interest.

Author details

Luke He[1,2], Ghufran S. Babar[1,3,4], Jacob M. Redel[3,4], Sabetha L. Young[5], Callie E. Chagas[5], Wayne V. Moore[1,3,4]* and Yun Yan[1,3,4]*

1 University of Missouri Kansas City, Kansas City, MO, USA

2 Department of Emergency Medicine, Creighton University, Phoenix, Arizona, USA

3 Department of Pediatrics, Division of Pediatric Endocrinology, Children's Mercy Kansas City, Kansas City, MO, USA

4 Children's Mercy Kansas City, Kansas City, MO, USA

5 Department of Nutrition, Children's Mercy Kansas City, Kansas City, MO, USA

*Address all correspondence to: yyan@cmh.edu and wmoore@cmh.edu

References

[1] Vos MB, Kimmons JE, Gillespie C, Welsh J, Blanck HM. Dietary fructose consumption among US children and adults: the Third National Health and Nutrition Examination Survey. Medscape journal of medicine. 2008; 10:160.

[2] Wang YC, Bleich SN, Gortmaker SL. Increasing caloric contribution from sugar-sweetened beverages and 100% fruit juices among US children and adolescents, 1988-2004. Pediatrics. 2008;121:e1604-14. DOI: 10.1542/peds.2007-2834.

[3] Marriott BP, Cole N, Lee E. National estimates of dietary fructose intake increased from 1977 to 2004 in the United States. The Journal of nutrition. 2009;139:1228S–35S. DOI: 10.3945/jn.108.098277.

[4] USDA. Dietary Guidelines for Americans 2015-2020, Eighth Edition. US Department of Health and Human Services. 2015.

[5] WHO. WHO calls on contries to reduce sugars intake among adults and children. 2015.

[6] Jegatheesan P, De Bandt JP. Fructose and NAFLD: The Multifaceted Aspects of Fructose Metabolism. Nutrients. 2017;9. DOI: 10.3390/nu9030230.

[7] Tran LT, Yuen VG, McNeill JH. The fructose-fed rat: a review on the mechanisms of fructose-induced insulin resistance and hypertension. Mol Cell Biochem. 2009;332:145-59. DOI: 10.1007/s11010-009-0184-4.

[8] Rippe JM, Angelopoulos TJ. Fructose-containing sugars and cardiovascular disease. Advances in nutrition. 2015;6:430-9. DOI: 10.3945/an.114.008177.

[9] Tappy L. Fructose-containing caloric sweeteners as a cause of obesity and metabolic disorders. J Exp Biol. 2018;221. DOI: 10.1242/jeb.164202.

[10] Bawden SJ, Stephenson MC, Ciampi E, Hunter K, Marciani L, Macdonald IA, et al. Investigating the effects of an oral fructose challenge on hepatic ATP reserves in healthy volunteers: A (31)P MRS study. Clin Nutr. 2016;35:645-9. DOI: 10.1016/j.clnu.2015.04.001.

[11] Bray GA. Energy and fructose from beverages sweetened with sugar or high-fructose corn syrup pose a health risk for some people. Advances in nutrition. 2013;4:220-5. DOI: 10.3945/an.112.002816.

[12] Tappy L, Rosset R. Health outcomes of a high fructose intake: the importance of physical activity. J Physiol. 2019;597:3561-71. DOI: 10.1113/JP278246.

[13] Softic S, Stanhope KL, Boucher J, Divanovic S, Lanaspa MA, Johnson RJ, et al. Fructose and hepatic insulin resistance. Crit Rev Clin Lab Sci. 2020;57:308-22. DOI: 10.1080/10408363.2019.1711360.

[14] Semnani-Azad Z, Khan TA, Blanco Mejia S, de Souza RJ, Leiter LA, Kendall CWC, et al. Association of Major Food Sources of Fructose-Containing Sugars With Incident Metabolic Syndrome: A Systematic Review and Meta-analysis. JAMA Netw Open. 2020;3:e209993. DOI: 10.1001/jamanetworkopen.2020.9993.

[15] Tappy L, Le KA. Metabolic effects of fructose and the worldwide increase in obesity. Physiol Rev. 2010;90:23-46. DOI: 10.1152/physrev.00019.2009.

[16] Karim S, Adams DH, Lalor PF. Hepatic expression and

cellular distribution of the glucose transporter family. World J Gastroenterol. 2012;18:6771-81. DOI: 10.3748/wjg.v18.i46.6771.

[17] Sun SZ, Empie MW. Fructose metabolism in humans - what isotopic tracer studies tell us. Nutrition & metabolism. 2012;9:89. DOI: 10.1186/1743-7075-9-89.

[18] Teff KL, Grudziak J, Townsend RR, Dunn TN, Grant RW, Adams SH, et al. Endocrine and metabolic effects of consuming fructose- and glucose-sweetened beverages with meals in obese men and women: influence of insulin resistance on plasma triglyceride responses. The Journal of clinical endocrinology and metabolism. 2009;94:1562-9. DOI: 10.1210/jc.2008-2192.

[19] Parniak MA, Kalant N. Enhancement of glycogen concentrations in primary cultures of rat hepatocytes exposed to glucose and fructose. Biochem J. 1988;251:795-802.

[20] Feinman RD, Fine EJ. Fructose in perspective. Nutrition & metabolism. 2013;10:45. DOI: 10.1186/1743-7075-10-45.

[21] Mayes PA. Intermediary metabolism of fructose. The American journal of clinical nutrition. 1993;58:754S–65S.

[22] Yan LJ. Redox imbalance stress in diabetes mellitus: Role of the polyol pathway. Animal Model Exp Med. 2018;1:7-13. DOI: 10.1002/ame2.12001.

[23] Lanaspa MA, Ishimoto T, Li N, Cicerchi C, Orlicky DJ, Ruzycki P, et al. Endogenous fructose production and metabolism in the liver contributes to the development of metabolic syndrome. Nat Commun. 2013;4:2434. DOI: 10.1038/ncomms3434.

[24] Behl T, Kaur I, Kotwani A. Implication of oxidative stress in progression of diabetic retinopathy. Surv Ophthalmol. 2016;61:187-96. DOI: 10.1016/j.survophthal.2015.06.001.

[25] Forbes JM, Coughlan MT, Cooper ME. Oxidative stress as a major culprit in kidney disease in diabetes. Diabetes. 2008;57:1446-54. DOI: 10.2337/db08-0057.

[26] Javed S, Petropoulos IN, Alam U, Malik RA. Treatment of painful diabetic neuropathy. Ther Adv Chronic Dis. 2015;6:15-28. DOI: 10.1177/2040622314552071.

[27] Brownlee M. Biochemistry and molecular cell biology of diabetic complications. Nature. 2001;414:813-20. DOI: 10.1038/414813a.

[28] Almenara CC, Mill JG, Vassallo DV, Baldo MP, Padilha AS. In vitro fructose exposure overactivates NADPH oxidase and causes oxidative stress in the isolated rat aorta. Toxicology in vitro : an international journal published in association with BIBRA. 2015;29:2030-7. DOI: 10.1016/j.tiv.2015.08.013.

[29] Leibowitz A, Rehman A, Paradis P, Schiffrin EL. Role of T regulatory lymphocytes in the pathogenesis of high-fructose diet-induced metabolic syndrome. Hypertension. 2013;61:1316-21. DOI: 10.1161/HYPERTENSIONAHA.111.203521.

[30] Litterio MC, Vazquez Prieto MA, Adamo AM, Elesgaray R, Oteiza PI, Galleano M, et al. (−)-Epicatechin reduces blood pressure increase in high-fructose-fed rats: effects on the determinants of nitric oxide bioavailability. J Nutr Biochem. 2015;26:745-51. DOI: 10.1016/j.jnutbio.2015.02.004.

[31] Glushakova O, Kosugi T, Roncal C, Mu W, Heinig M, Cirillo P, et al. Fructose induces the inflammatory molecule ICAM-1 in endothelial cells.

Journal of the American Society of Nephrology : JASN. 2008;19:1712-20. DOI: 10.1681/ASN.2007121304.

[32] Zhao CX, Xu X, Cui Y, Wang P, Wei X, Yang S, et al. Increased endothelial nitric-oxide synthase expression reduces hypertension and hyperinsulinemia in fructose-treated rats. The Journal of pharmacology and experimental therapeutics. 2009;328:610-20. DOI: 10.1124/jpet.108.143396.

[33] Romic S, Tepavcevic S, Zakula Z, Milosavljevic T, Stojiljkovic M, Zivkovic M, et al. Does oestradiol attenuate the damaging effects of a fructose-rich diet on cardiac Akt/endothelial nitric oxide synthase signalling? Br J Nutr. 2013;109:1940-8. DOI: 10.1017/S0007114512004114.

[34] Mattioli LF, Holloway NB, Thomas JH, Wood JG. Fructose, but not dextrose, induces leukocyte adherence to the mesenteric venule of the rat by oxidative stress. Pediatr Res. 2010;67:352-6.

[35] Schiano C, Grimaldi V, Franzese M, Fiorito C, De Nigris F, Donatelli F, et al. Non-nutritional sweeteners effects on endothelial vascular function. Toxicology in vitro : an international journal published in association with BIBRA. 2020;62:104694. DOI: 10.1016/j.tiv.2019.104694.

[36] Madero M, Perez-Pozo SE, Jalal D, Johnson RJ, Sanchez-Lozada LG. Dietary fructose and hypertension. Curr Hypertens Rep. 2011;13:29-35. DOI: 10.1007/s11906-010-0163-x.

[37] Perez-Pozo SE, Schold J, Nakagawa T, Sanchez-Lozada LG, Johnson RJ, Lillo JL. Excessive fructose intake induces the features of metabolic syndrome in healthy adult men: role of uric acid in the hypertensive response. International journal of obesity. 2010;34:454-61. DOI: 10.1038/ijo.2009.259.

[38] Brito JO, Ponciano K, Figueroa D, Bernardes N, Sanches IC, Irigoyen MC, et al. Parasympathetic dysfunction is associated with insulin resistance in fructose-fed female rats. Brazilian journal of medical and biological research = Revista brasileira de pesquisas medicas e biologicas. 2008;41:804-8.

[39] Jalal DI, Smits G, Johnson RJ, Chonchol M. Increased fructose associates with elevated blood pressure. Journal of the American Society of Nephrology : JASN. 2010;21:1543-9. DOI: 10.1681/ASN.2009111111.

[40] Fox IH, Kelley WN. Studies on the mechanism of fructose-induced hyperuricemia in man. Advances in experimental medicine and biology. 1974;41:463-70.

[41] Singh AK, Amlal H, Haas PJ, Dringenberg U, Fussell S, Barone SL, et al. Fructose-induced hypertension: essential role of chloride and fructose absorbing transporters PAT1 and Glut5. Kidney international. 2008;74:438-47. DOI: 10.1038/ki.2008.184.

[42] Xu C, Lu A, Lu X, Zhang L, Fang H, Zhou L, et al. Activation of Renal (Pro)Renin Receptor Contributes to High Fructose-Induced Salt Sensitivity. Hypertension. 2017;69:339-48. DOI: 10.1161/HYPERTENSIONAHA.116.08240.

[43] Oron-Herman M, Rosenthal T, Sela BA. Hyperhomocysteinemia as a component of syndrome X. Metabolism: clinical and experimental. 2003;52:1491-5.

[44] Tain YL, Lee WC, Leu S, Wu K, Chan J. High salt exacerbates programmed hypertension in maternal fructose-fed male offspring. Nutr Metab Cardiovasc Dis. 2015;25:1146-51. DOI: 10.1016/j.numecd.2015.08.002.

[45] Chan Q, Stamler J, Griep LM, Daviglus ML, Horn LV, Elliott P.

An Update on Nutrients and Blood Pressure. J Atheroscler Thromb. 2016;23:276-89. DOI: 10.5551/jat.30000.

[46] Chou CL, Pang CY, Lee TJ, Fang TC. Beneficial effects of calcitriol on hypertension, glucose intolerance, impairment of endothelium-dependent vascular relaxation, and visceral adiposity in fructose-fed hypertensive rats. PloS one. 2015;10:e0119843. DOI: 10.1371/journal.pone.0119843.

[47] Kelishadi R, Mansourian M, Heidari-Beni M. Association of fructose consumption and components of metabolic syndrome in human studies: a systematic review and meta-analysis. Nutrition. 2014;30:503-10. DOI: 10.1016/j.nut.2013.08.014.

[48] Brown CM, Dulloo AG, Yepuri G, Montani JP. Fructose ingestion acutely elevates blood pressure in healthy young humans. Am J Physiol Regul Integr Comp Physiol. 2008;294:R730-7. DOI: 10.1152/ajpregu.00680.2007.

[49] Chen L, Caballero B, Mitchell DC, Loria C, Lin PH, Champagne CM, et al. Reducing consumption of sugar-sweetened beverages is associated with reduced blood pressure: a prospective study among United States adults. Circulation. 2010;121:2398-406. DOI: 10.1161/CIRCULATIONAHA.109.911164.

[50] Saad AF, Dickerson J, Kechichian TB, Yin H, Gamble P, Salazar A, et al. High-fructose diet in pregnancy leads to fetal programming of hypertension, insulin resistance, and obesity in adult offspring. Am J Obstet Gynecol. 2016;215:378 e1-6. DOI: 10.1016/j.ajog.2016.03.038.

[51] Lanaspa MA, Kuwabara M, Andres-Hernando A, Li N, Cicerchi C, Jensen T, et al. High salt intake causes leptin resistance and obesity in mice by stimulating endogenous fructose production and metabolism. Proceedings of the National Academy of Sciences of the United States of America. 2018;115:3138-43. DOI: 10.1073/pnas.1713837115.

[52] Cai H, Li Z, Davis ME, Kanner W, Harrison DG, Dudley SC, Jr. Akt-dependent phosphorylation of serine 1179 and mitogen-activated protein kinase kinase/extracellular signal-regulated kinase 1/2 cooperatively mediate activation of the endothelial nitric-oxide synthase by hydrogen peroxide. Molecular pharmacology. 2003;63:325-31.

[53] Nakagawa T, Hu H, Zharikov S, Tuttle KR, Short RA, Glushakova O, et al. A causal role for uric acid in fructose-induced metabolic syndrome. American journal of physiology Renal physiology. 2006;290:F625-31. DOI: 10.1152/ajprenal.00140.2005.

[54] Choi YJ, Yoon Y, Lee KY, Hien TT, Kang KW, Kim KC, et al. Uric acid induces endothelial dysfunction by vascular insulin resistance associated with the impairment of nitric oxide synthesis. FASEB J. 2014;28:3197-204. DOI: 10.1096/fj.13-247148.

[55] Schwarz JM, Noworolski SM, Erkin-Cakmak A, Korn NJ, Wen MJ, Tai VW, et al. Effects of Dietary Fructose Restriction on Liver Fat, De Novo Lipogenesis, and Insulin Kinetics in Children With Obesity. Gastroenterology. 2017;153:743-52. DOI: 10.1053/j.gastro.2017.05.043.

[56] Dawber TR, Meadors GF, Moore FE, Jr. Epidemiological approaches to heart disease: the Framingham Study. Am J Public Health Nations Health. 1951;41:279-81.

[57] Abdel-Sayed A, Binnert C, Le KA, Bortolotti M, Schneiter P, Tappy L. A high-fructose diet impairs basal and stress-mediated lipid metabolism in healthy male subjects. The British journal of nutrition. 2008;100:393-9. DOI: 10.1017/S000711450789547X.

[58] Couchepin C, Le KA, Bortolotti M, da Encarnacao JA, Oboni JB, Tran C, et al. Markedly blunted metabolic effects of fructose in healthy young female subjects compared with male subjects. Diabetes Care. 2008;31:1254-6. DOI: 10.2337/dc07-2001.

[59] Leibowitz A, Rehman A, Paradis P, Schiffrin EL. Role of T regulatory lymphocytes in the pathogenesis of high-fructose diet-induced metabolic syndrome. Hypertension. 2013;61:1316-21.

[60] Stanhope KL, Schwarz JM, Keim NL, Griffen SC, Bremer AA, Graham JL, et al. Consuming fructose-sweetened, not glucose-sweetened, beverages increases visceral adiposity and lipids and decreases insulin sensitivity in overweight/obese humans. The Journal of clinical investigation. 2009;119:1322-34. DOI: 10.1172/JCI37385.

[61] Tappy L, Egli L, Lecoultre V, Schneider P. Effects of fructose-containing caloric sweeteners on resting energy expenditure and energy efficiency: a review of human trials. Nutr Metab (Lond). 2013;10:54. DOI: 10.1186/1743-7075-10-54.

[62] Dubois L, Farmer A, Girard M, Peterson K. Regular sugar-sweetened beverage consumption between meals increases risk of overweight among preschool-aged children. J Am Diet Assoc. 2007;107:924-34; discussion 34-5. DOI: 10.1016/j.jada.2007.03.004.

[63] Grummon AH, Smith NR, Golden SD, Frerichs L, Taillie LS, Brewer NT. Health Warnings on Sugar-Sweetened Beverages: Simulation of Impacts on Diet and Obesity Among U.S. Adults. Am J Prev Med. 2019;57:765-74. DOI: 10.1016/j.amepre.2019.06.022.

[64] Lim S, Zoellner JM, Lee JM, Burt BA, Sandretto AM, Sohn W, et al. Obesity and sugar-sweetened beverages in African-American preschool children: a longitudinal study. Obesity (Silver Spring). 2009;17:1262-8. DOI: 10.1038/oby.2008.656.

[65] Vinke PC, Blijleven KA, Luitjens M, Corpeleijn E. Young Children's Sugar-Sweetened Beverage Consumption and 5-Year Change in BMI: Lessons Learned from the Timing of Consumption. Nutrients. 2020;12. DOI: 10.3390/nu12082486.

[66] Vercammen KA, Frelier JM, Lowery CM, McGlone ME, Ebbeling CB, Bleich SN. A systematic review of strategies to reduce sugar-sweetened beverage consumption among 0-year to 5-year olds. Obes Rev. 2018;19:1504-24. DOI: 10.1111/obr.12741.

[67] Bray GA, Popkin BM. Dietary sugar and body weight: have we reached a crisis in the epidemic of obesity and diabetes?: health be damned! Pour on the sugar. Diabetes Care. 2014;37:950-6. DOI: 10.2337/dc13-2085.

[68] Zhang DM, Jiao RQ, Kong LD. High Dietary Fructose: Direct or Indirect Dangerous Factors Disturbing Tissue and Organ Functions. Nutrients. 2017;9. DOI: 10.3390/nu9040335.

[69] Golbahar J, Aminzadeh MA, Kassab SE, Omrani GR. Hyperhomocysteinemia induces insulin resistance in male Sprague-Dawley rats. Diabetes Res Clin Pract. 2007;76:1-5. DOI: 10.1016/j.diabres.2006.07.026.

[70] Spengler EK, Loomba R. Recommendations for Diagnosis, Referral for Liver Biopsy, and Treatment of Nonalcoholic Fatty Liver Disease and Nonalcoholic Steatohepatitis. Mayo Clin Proc. 2015;90:1233-46. DOI: 10.1016/j.mayocp.2015.06.013.

[71] Fusillo S, Rudolph B. Nonalcoholic fatty liver disease. Pediatr Rev. 2015;36:198-205; quiz 6. DOI: 10.1542/pir.36-5-198.

[72] Conlon BA, Beasley JM, Aebersold K, Jhangiani SS, Wylie-Rosett J. Nutritional management of insulin resistance in nonalcoholic fatty liver disease (NAFLD). Nutrients. 2013;5:4093-114. DOI: 10.3390/nu5104093.

[73] Jensen T, Abdelmalek MF, Sullivan S, Nadeau KJ, Green M, Roncal C, et al. Fructose and sugar: A major mediator of non-alcoholic fatty liver disease. J Hepatol. 2018;68:1063-75. DOI: 10.1016/j.jhep.2018.01.019.

[74] Crescenzo R, Bianco F, Falcone I, Coppola P, Liverini G, Iossa S. Increased hepatic de novo lipogenesis and mitochondrial efficiency in a model of obesity induced by diets rich in fructose. Eur J Nutr. 2013;52:537-45. DOI: 10.1007/s00394-012-0356-y.

[75] Renaud HJ, Cui JY, Lu H, Klaassen CD. Effect of diet on expression of genes involved in lipid metabolism, oxidative stress, and inflammation in mouse liver-insights into mechanisms of hepatic steatosis. PLoS One. 2014;9:e88584. DOI: 10.1371/journal.pone.0088584.

[76] Boesch C, Elsing C, Wegmuller H, Felblinger J, Vock P, Reichen J. Effect of ethanol and fructose on liver metabolism: a dynamic 31Phosphorus magnetic resonance spectroscopy study in normal volunteers. Magn Reson Imaging. 1997;15:1067-77.

[77] Latta M, Kunstle G, Lucas R, Hentze H, Wendel A. ATP-depleting carbohydrates prevent tumor necrosis factor receptor 1-dependent apoptotic and necrotic liver injury in mice. J Pharmacol Exp Ther. 2007;321:875-83. DOI: 10.1124/jpet.107.119958.

[78] Kanuri G, Spruss A, Wagnerberger S, Bischoff SC, Bergheim I. Role of tumor necrosis factor alpha (TNFalpha) in the onset of fructose-induced nonalcoholic fatty liver disease in mice. J Nutr Biochem. 2011;22:527-34. DOI: 10.1016/j.jnutbio.2010.04.007.

[79] Bray GA, Nielsen SJ, Popkin BM. Consumption of high-fructose corn syrup in beverages may play a role in the epidemic of obesity. The American journal of clinical nutrition. 2004;79:537-43.

[80] Vila L, Rebollo A, Adalsteisson GS, Alegret M, Merlos M, Roglans N, et al. Reduction of liver fructokinase expression and improved hepatic inflammation and metabolism in liquid fructose-fed rats after atorvastatin treatment. Toxicol Appl Pharmacol. 2011;251:32-40. DOI: 10.1016/j.taap.2010.11.011.

[81] Ter Horst KW, Serlie MJ. Fructose Consumption, Lipogenesis, and Non-Alcoholic Fatty Liver Disease. Nutrients. 2017;9. DOI: 10.3390/nu9090981.

[82] Softic S, Cohen DE, Kahn CR. Role of Dietary Fructose and Hepatic De Novo Lipogenesis in Fatty Liver Disease. Dig Dis Sci. 2016;61:1282-93. DOI: 10.1007/s10620-016-4054-0.

[83] Sapp V, Gaffney L, EauClaire SF, Matthews RP. Fructose leads to hepatic steatosis in zebrafish that is reversed by mechanistic target of rapamycin (mTOR) inhibition. Hepatology. 2014;60:1581-92. DOI: 10.1002/hep.27284.

[84] Yki-Jarvinen H. Nutritional modulation of nonalcoholic fatty liver disease and insulin resistance: human data. Curr Opin Clin Nutr Metab Care. 2010;13:709-14. DOI: 10.1097/MCO.0b013e32833f4b34.

[85] Schwarz JM, Noworolski SM, Wen MJ, Dyachenko A, Prior JL, Weinberg ME, et al. Effect of a High-Fructose Weight-Maintaining Diet on Lipogenesis and Liver Fat. J Clin

Endocrinol Metab. 2015;100:2434-42. DOI: 10.1210/jc.2014-3678.

[86] Chung M, Ma J, Patel K, Berger S, Lau J, Lichtenstein AH. Fructose, high-fructose corn syrup, sucrose, and nonalcoholic fatty liver disease or indexes of liver health: a systematic review and meta-analysis. The American journal of clinical nutrition. 2014;100:833-49. DOI: 10.3945/ajcn.114.086314.

[87] Nassir F, Ibdah JA. Sirtuins and nonalcoholic fatty liver disease. World J Gastroenterol. 2016;22:10084-92. DOI: 10.3748/wjg.v22.i46.10084.

[88] Guarente L. Sirtuins as potential targets for metabolic syndrome. Nature. 2006;444:868-74. DOI: 10.1038/nature05486.

[89] Rodgers JT, Lerin C, Haas W, Gygi SP, Spiegelman BM, Puigserver P. Nutrient control of glucose homeostasis through a complex of PGC-1alpha and SIRT1. Nature. 2005;434:113-8. DOI: 10.1038/nature03354.

[90] Sodhi K, Puri N, Favero G, Stevens S, Meadows C, Abraham NG, et al. Fructose Mediated Non-Alcoholic Fatty Liver Is Attenuated by HO-1-SIRT1 Module in Murine Hepatocytes and Mice Fed a High Fructose Diet. PloS one. 2015;10:e0128648. DOI: 10.1371/journal.pone.0128648.

[91] Yamazaki Y, Usui I, Kanatani Y, Matsuya Y, Tsuneyama K, Fujisaka S, et al. Treatment with SRT1720, a SIRT1 activator, ameliorates fatty liver with reduced expression of lipogenic enzymes in MSG mice. Am J Physiol Endocrinol Metab. 2009;297:E1179-86. DOI: 10.1152/ajpendo.90997.2008.

[92] Song YM, Lee YH, Kim JW, Ham DS, Kang ES, Cha BS, et al. Metformin alleviates hepatosteatosis by restoring SIRT1-mediated autophagy induction via an AMP-activated protein kinase-independent pathway. Autophagy. 2015;11:46-59. DOI: 10.4161/15548627.2014.984271.

[93] Kim TH, Yang YM, Han CY, Koo JH, Oh H, Kim SS, et al. Galpha12 ablation exacerbates liver steatosis and obesity by suppressing USP22/SIRT1-regulated mitochondrial respiration. The Journal of clinical investigation. 2018;128:5587-602. DOI: 10.1172/JCI97831.

[94] Martins IJ. Induction of NAFLD with Increased Risk of Obesity and Chronic Diseases in Developed Countrries. Open Journal of Endocrine and Metabolic Diseases. 2014;4:21. DOI: 10.4236/ojemd.2014.44011.

[95] Martins IJ. Nutrition Therapy Regulates Caffeine Metabolism with Relevance to NaflD and Induction of Type 3 Diabetes. HSOA Journal of Diabetes and Metabolic Disorders 2017;4:10. DOI: 10.24966/DMD-201X/100019.

[96] Rebollo A, Roglans N, Baena M. Liquid fructose downregulates Sirt1 expression and activity and impairs the oxidation of fatty acids in rat and human liver cells. Biochim Biophys Acta. 2014;1841:514-24.

[97] Chen XY, Cai CZ, Yu ML, Feng ZM, Zhang YW, Liu PH, et al. LB100 ameliorates nonalcoholic fatty liver disease via the AMPK/Sirt1 pathway. World J Gastroenterol. 2019;25:6607-18. DOI: 10.3748/wjg.v25.i45.6607.

[98] Carafa V, Rotili D, Forgione M, Cuomo F, Serretiello E, Hailu GS, et al. Sirtuin functions and modulation: from chemistry to the clinic. Clin Epigenetics. 2016;8:61. DOI: 10.1186/s13148-016-0224-3.

[99] Colak Y, Yesil A, Mutlu HH, Caklili OT, Ulasoglu C, Senates E, et al. A potential treatment of non-alcoholic fatty liver disease with SIRT1 activators.

J Gastrointestin Liver Dis. 2014;23:311-9. DOI: 10.15403/jgld.2014.1121.233.yck.

[100] Stanisic J, Koricanac G, Culafic T, Romic S, Stojiljkovic M, Kostic M, et al. Low intensity exercise prevents disturbances in rat cardiac insulin signaling and endothelial nitric oxide synthase induced by high fructose diet. Molecular and cellular endocrinology. 2016;420:97-104. DOI: 10.1016/j.mce.2015.11.032.

[101] Hwang IS, Ho H, Hoffman BB, Reaven GM. Fructose-induced insulin resistance and hypertension in rats. Hypertension. 1987;10:512-6. DOI: 10.1161/01.hyp.10.5.512.

[102] Jenkins DJ, Wolever TM, Buckley G, Lam KY, Giudici S, Kalmusky J, et al. Low-glycemic-index starchy foods in the diabetic diet. The American journal of clinical nutrition. 1988;48:248-54.

[103] Wu T, Giovannucci E, Pischon T, Hankinson SE, Ma J, Rifai N, et al. Fructose, glycemic load, and quantity and quality of carbohydrate in relation to plasma C-peptide concentrations in US women. The American journal of clinical nutrition. 2004;80:1043-9.

[104] Shulga N, Pastorino JG. Fructose sensitizes pancreatic beta cells to TNFalpha-induced necroptosis. Biol Open. 2015. DOI: 10.1242/bio.014712.

[105] Zakula Z, Koricanac G, Tepavcevic S, Stojiljkovic M, Milosavljevic T, Isenovic ER. Impairment of cardiac insulin signaling in fructose-fed ovariectomized female Wistar rats. European journal of nutrition. 2011;50:543-51. DOI: 10.1007/s00394-010-0161-4.

[106] Belosludtsev KN, Belosludtseva NV, Dubinin MV. Diabetes Mellitus, Mitochondrial Dysfunction and Ca(2+)-Dependent Permeability Transition Pore. Int J Mol Sci. 2020;21. DOI: 10.3390/ijms21186559.

[107] Fujimoto K, Chen Y, Polonsky KS, Dorn GW, 2nd. Targeting cyclophilin D and the mitochondrial permeability transition enhances beta-cell survival and prevents diabetes in Pdx1 deficiency. Proceedings of the National Academy of Sciences of the United States of America. 2010;107:10214-9. DOI: 10.1073/pnas.0914209107.

[108] Lablanche S, Cottet-Rousselle C, Lamarche F, Benhamou PY, Halimi S, Leverve X, et al. Protection of pancreatic INS-1 beta-cells from glucose- and fructose-induced cell death by inhibiting mitochondrial permeability transition with cyclosporin A or metformin. Cell death & disease. 2011;2:e134. DOI: 10.1038/cddis.2011.15.

[109] Mitrakou A, Kelley D, Veneman T, Jenssen T, Pangburn T, Reilly J, et al. Contribution of abnormal muscle and liver glucose metabolism to postprandial hyperglycemia in NIDDM. Diabetes. 1990;39:1381-90.

[110] Matschinsky FM. Glucokinase as glucose sensor and metabolic signal generator in pancreatic beta-cells and hepatocytes. Diabetes. 1990;39:647-52.

[111] Rossetti L, Giaccari A, Barzilai N, Howard K, Sebel G, Hu M. Mechanism by which hyperglycemia inhibits hepatic glucose production in conscious rats. Implications for the pathophysiology of fasting hyperglycemia in diabetes. The Journal of clinical investigation. 1993;92:1126-34. DOI: 10.1172/JCI116681.

[112] Shiota M, Galassetti P, Monohan M, Neal DW, Cherrington AD. Small amounts of fructose markedly augment net hepatic glucose uptake in the conscious dog. Diabetes. 1998;47:867-73.

[113] Agius L, Peak M, Newgard CB, Gomez-Foix AM, Guinovart JJ. Evidence

for a role of glucose-induced translocation of glucokinase in the control of hepatic glycogen synthesis. The Journal of biological chemistry. 1996;271:30479-86.

[114] Kim M, Do GY, Kim I. Activation of the renin-angiotensin system in high fructose-induced metabolic syndrome. Korean J Physiol Pharmacol. 2020;24:319-28. DOI: 10.4196/kjpp.2020.24.4.319.

[115] Petersen KF, Laurent D, Yu C, Cline GW, Shulman GI. Stimulating effects of low-dose fructose on insulin-stimulated hepatic glycogen synthesis in humans. Diabetes. 2001;50:1263-8.

[116] Gonzalez JT, Fuchs CJ, Betts JA, van Loon LJ. Liver glycogen metabolism during and after prolonged endurance-type exercise. Am J Physiol Endocrinol Metab. 2016;311:E543-53. DOI: 10.1152/ajpendo.00232.2016.

[117] Lee JS, Jun DW, Kim EK, Jeon HJ, Nam HH, Saeed WK. Histologic and Metabolic Derangement in High-Fat, High-Fructose, and Combination Diet Animal Models. ScientificWorldJournal. 2015;2015:306326. DOI: 10.1155/2015/306326.

[118] Pyo YH, Lee KW. Preventive effect of Monascus-fermented products enriched with ubiquinones on type 2 diabetic rats induced by a high-fructose plus high-fat diet. J Med Food. 2014;17:826-9. DOI: 10.1089/jmf.2013.3001.

[119] Stark AH, Timar B, Madar Z. Adaptation of Sprague Dawley rats to long-term feeding of high fat or high fructose diets. European journal of nutrition. 2000;39:229-34. DOI: 10.1007/s003940070016.

[120] Wilson RD, Islam MS. Fructose-fed streptozotocin-injected rat: an alternative model for type 2 diabetes. Pharmacol Rep. 2012;64:129-39. DOI: 10.1016/s1734-1140(12)70739-9.

[121] Johnson RJ, Nakagawa T, Sanchez-Lozada LG, Shafiu M, Sundaram S, Le M, et al. Sugar, uric acid, and the etiology of diabetes and obesity. Diabetes. 2013;62:3307-15. DOI: 10.2337/db12-1814.

[122] DiNicolantonio JJ, O'Keefe JH, Lucan SC. Added fructose: a principal driver of type 2 diabetes mellitus and its consequences. Mayo Clin Proc. 2015;90:372-81. DOI: 10.1016/j.mayocp.2014.12.019.

[123] Malik VS, Hu FB. Fructose and Cardiometabolic Health: What the Evidence From Sugar-Sweetened Beverages Tells Us. J Am Coll Cardiol. 2015;66:1615-24. DOI: 10.1016/j.jacc.2015.08.025.

[124] Zheng J, Feng Q, Zhang Q, Wang T, Xiao X. Early Life Fructose Exposure and Its Implications for Long-Term Cardiometabolic Health in Offspring. Nutrients. 2016;8. DOI: 10.3390/nu8110685.

[125] Barriere DA, Noll C, Roussy G, Lizotte F, Kessai A, Kirby K, et al. Combination of high-fat/high-fructose diet and low-dose streptozotocin to model long-term type-2 diabetes complications. Sci Rep. 2018;8:424. DOI: 10.1038/s41598-017-18896-5.

[126] Kuzma JN, Cromer G, Hagman DK, Breymeyer KL, Roth CL, Foster-Schubert KE, et al. Consuming glucose-sweetened, not fructose-sweetened, beverages increases fasting insulin in healthy humans. Eur J Clin Nutr. 2019;73:487-90. DOI: 10.1038/s41430-018-0297-5.

[127] Hawkins M, Gabriely I, Wozniak R, Vilcu C, Shamoon H, Rossetti L. Fructose improves the ability of hyperglycemia per se to regulate glucose production

in type 2 diabetes. Diabetes. 2002;51:606-14.

[128] Dornas WC, de Lima WG, Pedrosa ML, Silva ME. Health implications of high-fructose intake and current research. Advances in nutrition. 2015;6:729-37. DOI: 10.3945/an.114.008144.

[129] Wang DD, Sievenpiper JL, de Souza RJ, Chiavaroli L, Ha V, Cozma AI, et al. The effects of fructose intake on serum uric acid vary among controlled dietary trials. The Journal of nutrition. 2012;142:916-23. DOI: 10.3945/jn.111.151951.

[130] DeBosch BJ, Chen Z, Finck BN, Chi M, Moley KH. Glucose transporter-8 (GLUT8) mediates glucose intolerance and dyslipidemia in high-fructose diet-fed male mice. Molecular endocrinology. 2013;27:1887-96. DOI: 10.1210/me.2013-1137.

[131] Bode JC, Zelder O, Rumpelt HJ, Wittkamp U. Depletion of liver adenosine phosphates and metabolic effects of intravenous infusion of fructose or sorbitol in man and in the rat. Eur J Clin Invest. 1973;3:436-41. DOI: 10.1111/j.1365-2362.1973.tb02211.x.

[132] Rho YH, Zhu Y, Choi HK. The epidemiology of uric acid and fructose. Semin Nephrol. 2011;31:410-9. DOI: 10.1016/j.semnephrol.2011.08.004.

[133] Sayehmiri K, Ahmadi I, Anvari E. Fructose Feeding and Hyperuricemia: a Systematic Review and Meta-Analysis. Clin Nutr Res. 2020;9:122-33. DOI: 10.7762/cnr.2020.9.2.122.

[134] Ebrahimpour-Koujan S, Saneei P, Larijani B, Esmaillzadeh A. Consumption of sugar-sweetened beverages and serum uric acid concentrations: a systematic review and meta-analysis. J Hum Nutr Diet. 2020. DOI: 10.1111/jhn.12796.

[135] Schwingshackl L, Neuenschwander M, Hoffmann G, Buyken AE, Schlesinger S. Dietary sugars and cardiometabolic risk factors: a network meta-analysis on isocaloric substitution interventions. The American journal of clinical nutrition. 2020;111:187-96. DOI: 10.1093/ajcn/nqz273.

[136] Kusuhara S, Fukushima Y, Ogura S, Inoue N, Uemura A. Pathophysiology of Diabetic Retinopathy: The Old and the New. Diabetes Metab J. 2018;42:364-76. DOI: 10.4093/dmj.2018.0182.

[137] Kearney FM, Fagan XJ, Al-Qureshi S. Review of the role of refined dietary sugars (fructose and glucose) in the genesis of retinal disease. Clin Experiment Ophthalmol. 2014;42:564-73. DOI: 10.1371/journal.pone.0112450.

[138] Thierry M, Pasquis B, Acar N, Gregoire S, Febvret V, Buteau B, et al. Metabolic syndrome triggered by high-fructose diet favors choroidal neovascularization and impairs retinal light sensitivity in the rat. PloS one. 2014;9:e112450. DOI: 10.1371/journal.pone.0112450.

[139] Vidal E, Lalarme E, Maire MA, Febvret V, Gregoire S, Gambert S, et al. Early impairments in the retina of rats fed with high fructose/high fat diet are associated with glucose metabolism deregulation but not dyslipidaemia. Sci Rep. 2019;9:5997. DOI: 10.1038/s41598-019-42528-9.

[140] Lutty GA. Effects of diabetes on the eye. Invest Ophthalmol Vis Sci. 2013;54:ORSF81-7. DOI: 10.1167/iovs.13-12979.

[141] Besharse JC, Dunis DA. Methoxyindoles and photoreceptor metabolism: activation of rod shedding. Science. 1983;219:1341-3.

[142] Pierce ME, Besharse JC. Melatonin and rhythmic photoreceptor

metabolism: melatonin-induced cone elongation is blocked at high light intensity. Brain Res. 1987;405:400-4.

[143] Osborne NN, Nash MS, Wood JP. Melatonin counteracts ischemia-induced apoptosis in human retinal pigment epithelial cells. Invest Ophthalmol Vis Sci. 1998;39:2374-83.

[144] Valenzuela-Melgarejo FJ, Caro-Diaz C, Cabello-Guzman G. Potential Crosstalk between Fructose and Melatonin: A New Role of Melatonin-Inhibiting the Metabolic Effects of Fructose. Int J Endocrinol. 2018;2018:7515767. DOI: 10.1155/2018/7515767.

[145] Pourhanifeh MH, Hosseinzadeh A, Dehdashtian E, Hemati K, Mehrzadi S. Melatonin: new insights on its therapeutic properties in diabetic complications. Diabetol Metab Syndr. 2020;12:30. DOI: 10.1186/s13098-020-00537-z.

[146] Stitt AW, Hughes SJ, Canning P, Lynch O, Cox O, Frizzell N, et al. Substrates modified by advanced glycation end-products cause dysfunction and death in retinal pericytes by reducing survival signals mediated by platelet-derived growth factor. Diabetologia. 2004;47:1735-46. DOI: 10.1007/s00125-004-1523-3.

[147] Nishikawa T, Edelstein D, Brownlee M. The missing link: a single unifying mechanism for diabetic complications. Kidney Int Suppl. 2000;77:S26-30.

[148] Yerneni KK, Bai W, Khan BV, Medford RM, Natarajan R. Hyperglycemia-induced activation of nuclear transcription factor kappaB in vascular smooth muscle cells. Diabetes. 1999;48:855-64.

[149] Donnelly R, Idris I, Forrester JV. Protein kinase C inhibition and diabetic retinopathy: a shot in the dark at translational research. Br J Ophthalmol. 2004;88:145-51. DOI: 10.1136/bjo.88.1.145.

[150] Nakagawa T, Lanaspa MA, Millan IS, Fini M, Rivard CJ, Sanchez-Lozada LG, et al. Fructose contributes to the Warburg effect for cancer growth. Cancer Metab. 2020;8:16. DOI: 10.1186/s40170-020-00222-9.

[151] Segditsas S, Rowan AJ, Howarth K, Jones A, Leedham S, Wright NA, et al. APC and the three-hit hypothesis. Oncogene. 2009;28:146-55. DOI: 10.1038/onc.2008.361.

[152] Santhekadur PK. The dark face of fructose as a tumor promoter. Genes Dis. 2020;7:163-5. DOI: 10.1016/j.gendis.2019.10.001.

[153] Mahraoui L, Rousset M, Dussaulx E, Darmoul D, Zweibaum A, Brot-Laroche E. Expression and localization of GLUT-5 in Caco-2 cells, human small intestine, and colon. The American journal of physiology. 1992;263:G312-8. DOI: 10.1152/ajpgi.1992.263.3.G312.

[154] Zamora-Leon SP, Golde DW, Concha, II, Rivas CI, Delgado-Lopez F, Baselga J, et al. Expression of the fructose transporter GLUT5 in human breast cancer. Proceedings of the National Academy of Sciences of the United States of America. 1996;93:1847-52. DOI: 10.1073/pnas.93.5.1847.

[155] Feng CY, Wong S, Dong Q, Bruce J, Mehta R, Bruce WR, et al. Hepatocyte inflammation model for cytotoxicity research: fructose or glycolaldehyde as a source of endogenous toxins. Arch Physiol Biochem. 2009;115:105-11. DOI: 10.1080/13813450902887055.

[156] Svendsen C, Hoie AH, Alexander J, Murkovic M, Husoy T. The food processing contaminant glyoxal promotes tumour growth in the multiple

intestinal neoplasia (Min) mouse model. Food Chem Toxicol. 2016;94:197-202. DOI: 10.1016/j.fct.2016.06.006.

[157] Goncalves MD, Lu C, Tutnauer J, Hartman TE, Hwang SK, Murphy CJ, et al. High-fructose corn syrup enhances intestinal tumor growth in mice. Science. 2019;363:1345-9. DOI: 10.1126/science.aat8515.

[158] Yalcin A, Telang S, Clem B, Chesney J. Regulation of glucose metabolism by 6-phosphofructo-2-kinase/fructose-2,6-bisphosphatases in cancer. Exp Mol Pathol. 2009;86:174-9. DOI: 10.1016/j.yexmp.2009.01.003.

[159] Charrez B, Qiao L, Hebbard L. The role of fructose in metabolism and cancer. Horm Mol Biol Clin Investig. 2015;22:79-89. DOI: 10.1515/hmbci-2015-0009.

[160] San-Millan I, Brooks GA. Reexamining cancer metabolism: lactate production for carcinogenesis could be the purpose and explanation of the Warburg Effect. Carcinogenesis. 2017;38:119-33. DOI: 10.1093/carcin/bgw127.

[161] Brizel DM, Schroeder T, Scher RL, Walenta S, Clough RW, Dewhirst MW, et al. Elevated tumor lactate concentrations predict for an increased risk of metastases in head-and-neck cancer. Int J Radiat Oncol Biol Phys. 2001;51:349-53. DOI: 10.1016/s0360-3016(01)01630-3.

[162] Kumar VB, Viji RI, Kiran MS, Sudhakaran PR. Endothelial cell response to lactate: implication of PAR modification of VEGF. J Cell Physiol. 2007;211:477-85. DOI: 10.1002/jcp.20955.

[163] Vegran F, Boidot R, Michiels C, Sonveaux P, Feron O. Lactate influx through the endothelial cell monocarboxylate transporter MCT1 supports an NF-kappaB/IL-8 pathway that drives tumor angiogenesis. Cancer Res. 2011;71:2550-60. DOI: 10.1158/0008-5472.CAN-10-2828.

[164] Lanaspa MA, Sanchez-Lozada LG, Choi YJ, Cicerchi C, Kanbay M, Roncal-Jimenez CA, et al. Uric acid induces hepatic steatosis by generation of mitochondrial oxidative stress: potential role in fructose-dependent and -independent fatty liver. The Journal of biological chemistry. 2012;287:40732-44. DOI: 10.1074/jbc.M112.399899.

[165] Weinberg F, Hamanaka R, Wheaton WW, Weinberg S, Joseph J, Lopez M, et al. Mitochondrial metabolism and ROS generation are essential for Kras-mediated tumorigenicity. Proceedings of the National Academy of Sciences of the United States of America. 2010;107:8788-93. DOI: 10.1073/pnas.1003428107.

[166] Brown JM, Wilson WR. Exploiting tumour hypoxia in cancer treatment. Nat Rev Cancer. 2004;4:437-47. DOI: 10.1038/nrc1367.

[167] Hood K, Hollaway MR. The significant role of fructose-1,6-diphosphate in the regulatory kinetics of phosphofructokinase. FEBS Lett. 1976;68:8-14. DOI: 10.1016/0014-5793(76)80392-4.

[168] Monzavi-Karbassi B, Hine RJ, Stanley JS, Ramani VP, Carcel-Trullols J, Whitehead TL, et al. Fructose as a carbon source induces an aggressive phenotype in MDA-MB-468 breast tumor cells. Int J Oncol. 2010;37:615-22. DOI: 10.3892/ijo_00000710.

[169] Jiang Y, Pan Y, Rhea PR, Tan L, Gagea M, Cohen L, et al. A Sucrose-Enriched Diet Promotes Tumorigenesis in Mammary Gland in Part through the 12-Lipoxygenase Pathway. Cancer Res. 2016;76:24-9. DOI: 10.1158/0008-5472.CAN-14-3432.

[170] Strober JW, Brady MJ. Dietary Fructose Consumption and Triple-Negative Breast Cancer Incidence. Front Endocrinol (Lausanne). 2019;10:367. DOI: 10.3389/fendo.2019.00367.

[171] Liu H, Huang D, McArthur DL, Boros LG, Nissen N, Heaney AP. Fructose induces transketolase flux to promote pancreatic cancer growth. Cancer Res. 2010;70:6368-76. DOI: 10.1158/0008-5472.CAN-09-4615.

[172] Carreno D, Corro N, Torres-Estay V, Veliz LP, Jaimovich R, Cisternas P, et al. Fructose and prostate cancer: toward an integrated view of cancer cell metabolism. Prostate Cancer Prostatic Dis. 2019;22:49-58. DOI: 10.1038/s41391-018-0072-7.

[173] Hers HG. [The mechanism of the formation of seminal fructose and fetal fructose]. Biochim Biophys Acta. 1960;37:127-38. DOI: 10.1016/0006-3002(60)90086-x.

[174] Saraswat M, Mrudula T, Kumar PU, Suneetha A, Rao Rao TS, Srinivasulu M, et al. Overexpression of aldose reductase in human cancer tissues. Med Sci Monit. 2006;12:CR525-9.

[175] Kranhold JF, Loh D, Morris RC, Jr. Renal fructose-metabolizing enzymes: significance in hereditary fructose intolerance. Science. 1969;165:402-3. DOI: 10.1126/science.165.3891.402.

Chapter 8

Main Organs Involved in Glucose Metabolism

Laura Lema-Pérez

Abstract

Sugar, or technically known as glucose, is the main source of energy of all cells in the human body. The glucose homeostasis cycle is the mechanism to maintain blood glucose levels in a healthy threshold. When this natural mechanism is broken, many metabolic disorders appear such as diabetes mellitus, and some substances of interest, like glucose, are out of control. In the mechanism to maintain blood glucose, several organs are involved but the role of most of them has been disregarded in the literature. In this chapter, the main organs involved in such a mechanism and their role in glucose metabolism are described. Specifically, the stomach and small intestine, organs of the gastrointestinal system, are the first to play an important role in the regulatory system, because it is where carbohydrates are digested and absorbed as glucose into the bloodstream. Then glucose as a simple substance goes to the liver to be stored as glycogen. Glucose storage occurs due to the delivery of hormones from the pancreas, which produces, stores, and releases insulin and glucagon, two antagonistic hormones with an important role in glucose metabolism. The kidneys assist the liver in insulin clearance in the postprandial state and gluconeogenesis in the post absorptive state. Physiological aspects and the detailed role of every organ involved in glucose metabolism are described in this chapter.

Keywords: glucose metabolism, homeostasis, diabetes mellitus

1. Introduction

Glucose is contained in foods rich in carbohydrates like bread, potatoes, rice, and fruits. It can be as a simple molecule, sugar, or complex molecules, carbohydrates. Although carbohydrates are more abundant in the diet, they are digested to be converted into glucose molecules to be absorbed in the gut. Previously to be absorbed, stomach and small intestine play an important role in digestion every particle ingested. First, food reaches the stomach after being chewed and swallowed from mouth. The digestion of carbohydrates begins in the mouth with saliva while chewing, but continues in the small intestine because the acidic pH of the stomach inactivates the amylase enzyme that is responsible for breaking them down. In the small intestine, the digestion of carbohydrates ends to be absorbed, through the enterocytes, into the blood. Once the glucose molecules are absorbed into the bloodstream, they reach the liver by traveling through the portal system. In the liver, they are partially stored as glycogen by the action of the insulin previously released in the pancreas. The rest of the glucose continues in the circulation, reaches the heart and all tissues and organs. Insulin concentrations are proportional to glucose concentrations due to this hormone make enter the glucose into the cells. In fact, insulin

IntechOpen

concentrations released by the pancreas are usually higher than glucose concentrations in blood. In this sense, the kidneys regulate glucose and insulin concentrations once these molecules reach them. Insulin is clearance in both, liver and kidneys, while glucose is produced from non-carbohydrates precursors in the postprandial state to compensate for the insulin excess in the blood. On the other hand, during a fasting period or a post-absorptive state, glucagon is released into the bloodstream by the pancreas and achieves the liver to dephosphorylate the glycogen into glucose to keep blood glucose levels in the healthy threshold. As can be seen from everything mentioned above, blood glucose levels can be set at the desired threshold thanks to the joint work between all the organs of the human body, where they all play an important role in this regulatory system. Next sections.

2. Importance of glucose in the human body

Cells of the tissues in the human body use glucose, the simplest of the carbohydrates, as the main source of energy to carry out their metabolic processes. Despite this, glucose consumption should be moderate because an excess can trigger multiple metabolic disorders that can even be chronic. Carbohydrates start to be processed immediately they are ingested, i.e., its digestion begins in the mouth with the amylase in the saliva. Then, ingested food travels throughout the esophagus to the stomach. In the stomach, the enzyme amylase is inactivated due to acidic pH, so carbohydrates cannot continue to digest. Other nutrients such as protein and fat are partially digested in the stomach, about 5% and 20%, respectively [1]. Once the ingested food has the appropriate rheological properties, it passes through the pylorus to reach the duodenum, the first part of the small intestine. In the duodenum, the bile produced from and gallbladder, is released to digest fats. The digestion of all nutrients ends in the small intestine by an additional intervention of the pancreas with the release of both pancreatic enzymes such as amylases, lipases, and proteases, and hormones such as insulin and glucagon. The molecules produced during digestion are absorbed by the enterocytes into the bloodstream. The rest of the food that is not absorbed in the small intestine passes into the colon.

Once glucose is in the systemic circulation, insulin hormone helps it to enter into the cells. Inside the cells, glucose is broken down to produce adenosine triphosphate (ATP) molecules by means of glycolysis. ATP are energy-rich molecules that power numerous cellular processes. Therefore, a constant supply of glucose from the blood to the cells must be ensured. Negative feedback systems [2] are responsible to ensure blood glucose concentrations in a normal range of 70 to 110 milligrams of glucose per deciliter of blood (mg / dL) [3]. Negative feedback systems are mechanisms that perceive changes in the human body and activate mechanisms that reverse the changes to restore conditions to their normal levels. Furthermore, negative feedback systems are critically important in glucose homeostasis in the maintenance of relatively constant internal conditions. In this regard, negative feedback systems make the pancreas to produce and release more insulin when there is an excess glucose consumption. This fact, maintained over time, can cause disruptions in glucose homeostasis lead to potentially life-threatening such as insulin resistance and diabetes mellitus.

The body also use other sources of energy such as amino acids (building blocks of proteins) and fats. However, despite these alternative energy sources, a minimum level of glucose in the blood must be ensured mainly for the metabolic activities of the brain and nervous system. Glucose is the main source of fuel for the brain and nervous system. Nerve cells and chemical messengers need glucose to process information. On the other hand, the liver and muscles can store the leftover glucose in little bundles called glycogen once the human body has used all the energy it needs. Glycogen works as a reserve fuel to be used during post-absorptive or fasting periods. Glycogenolysis is the biochemical process for converting glycogen to glucose in the liver. This process, together with the absorption of glucose in the small intestine after an ingested meal and the hepatic and renal gluconeogenesis, are the main factors to increase the levels of glucose in the blood. Sometimes, glucose levels in the blood can also go sky high under stressful conditions. Also, the High-Intensity Interval Training (HIIT) type of exercise is acknowledged to trigger (not completely understood) mechanisms able to rise the blood glucose levels. Contrary, the transport of the glucose into the cells by insulin action, physical exercise, and sometimes glycosuria (a condition characterized by an excess of sugar in the urine occurring under abnormal events when glucose homeostasis is impaired) are the main factors able to decrease blood glucose levels.

Regardless of the condition, the human body is designed to keep the level of glucose in the bloodstream in healthy levels. However, when the glucose homeostasis is broken, diseases such as diabetes mellitus appear and persistent high blood glucose can lead generating acute complications such as diabetic ketoacidosis, retinopathy, diabetic nephropathy, neuropathy, and cardio-cerebrovascular disease. How does the body for regulating glucose levels in the blood? The next section introduces the glucose regulation cycle in detail and the role of every organ that is involved.

3. The glucose regulation cycle

Glucose homeostasis is the mechanism able to maintain the blood glucose levels near the range of $70mg / dl$ to $110mg / dL$ by the action of a complex interplay among organs, hormones, metabolic-systems, and neural control mechanisms. As mentioned above, glucose is the main source of energy by allowing essential cellular processes such as respiration, tissue repair, cell multiplication, to be carried out, among others. Production and release of pancreatic hormones, mainly insulin and glucagon, ensures the glucose regulation in the blood [3]. **Figure 1** shows how the human body maintains glucose levels in a specific physiological range. Once carbohydrates nutrients are ingested and enter the digestive tube, several enzymes begin to work to digest macronutrients, e.g., amylases trigger for polysaccharide breakdown. In this way, polysaccharides are converted into monosaccharides, smaller molecules able to be absorbed by enterocytes in the small intestine. Monosaccharides absorption leads to increased blood glucose levels in the bloodstream. Simultaneously to this process, the incretin effect also occurs in which β-cells in the pancreas are stimulated by the action of GIP and GLP-1 hormones. Stimulation of β-cells drives the production and release of insulin, which increases the amount of GLUT4 glucose transporters in the cell membranes of different tissues [3]. Blood glucose concentrations also stimulate insulin production, and the hormones GIP and GLP-1 modulate it. As mentioned before, there are specialized molecules called GLUT to transport glucose from the blood into cells through cell membranes by diffusion. In this way, Excess glucose is eliminated from the blood, decreasing it. This process is represented in the figure with the plus sign. Therefore, glucose is transported within muscle and adipocytes cells, hepatocytes, neurons, etc., to be used as a source of energy. The liver is also answerable to sense blood glucose concentrations coming from the portal system and systemic circulation. In the liver, enzymes known as glucokinase are responsible to sense glucose amount, stimulate its diffusion through the hepatocytes, and simultaneously produce glycogen from glucose excess. Glycogen is a multibranched polysaccharide of glucose used as glucose storage to be used during fasting periods as an energy source in the cells [4].

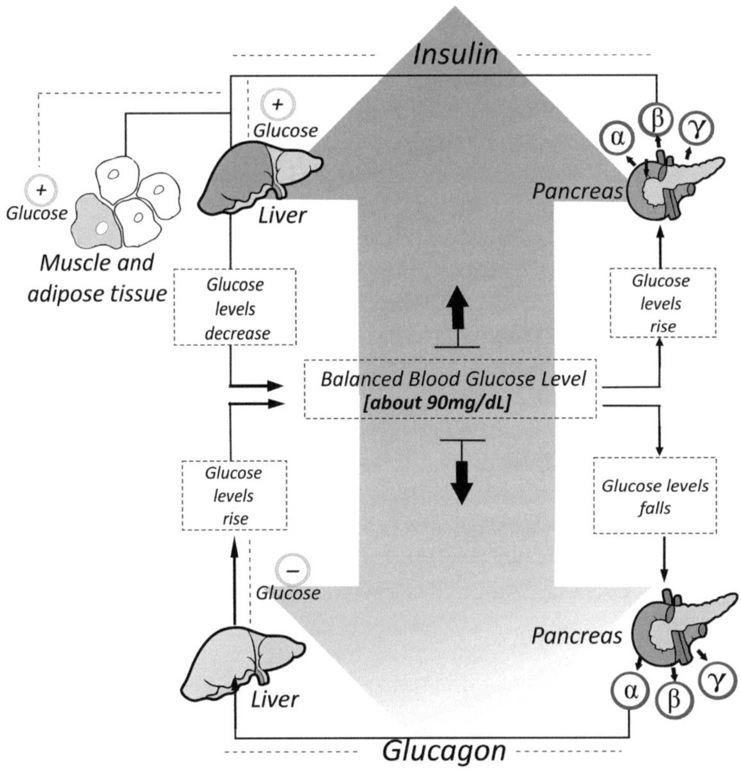

Figure 1.
The glucose homeostasis in the human body.

During fasting periods, glucose levels in the blood decrease causing inhibition of insulin production in the pancreas by the action of hormones known as catecholamines [4]. Consequently, α-cells in the pancreas are stimulated to produce glucagon hormone that acts antagonistically to insulin. Glucagon makes a function on the different hepatocyte receptors triggering both the action of the phosphorylase enzyme and the glycogenolysis process. Glycogenolysis is the process in which glycogen is converted into glucose to increase blood glucose levels and recover the lack of glucose, setting its concentrations in the desired levels [5]. This is symbolized in **Figure 1** by the minus sign.

Diabetes Mellitus is a condition appearing when the glucose homeostasis is broken, that is, plasma glucose levels are no longer maintained at desired levels. This is mainly due to a deficit in the production of insulin from the pancreatic β-cells or from a resistance to the action of the produced insulin.

4. Main organs involved in glucose homeostasis

Although some organs need fatty acids to carry out their metabolic processes, most tissues in the human body use glucose as their main source of energy. Good glucose utilization depends on keeping blood glucose levels within range at all times and on the proper functioning of the glucose homeostatic mechanism. Several complementary physiological processes are involved in the glucose homeostatic mechanism. The gastrointestinal tract is responsible to produce and absorb glucose, the liver carries out biochemical reactions such as glycogenolysis, glycolysis, and gluconeogenesis, the kidneys filter, reabsorb, and in some cases excrete glucose, and they also produce glucose from non-carbohydrate precursors. The role of the main organs involved in the glucose regulation cycle is described below.

4.1 Pancreas

The pancreas is a special organ because has both endocrine and exocrine functions. Exocrine functions consist of the production and secretion of digestive enzymes whereas endocrine functions include production and secretion of hormones. This chapter is primarily focused in the endocrine function given the crucial role on glucose homeostasis. Endocrine component of the pancreas consists of clustered cells forming the so-called islets of Langerhans. Islets of Langerhans are small island-shaped structures within exocrine pancreatic tissue representing only 1–2% of the entire organ [6]. The pancreatic islet endocrine cells include five different types that produce and release important hormones directly into the bloodstream: α -cells produce glucagon, β -cells produce amylin-, C-peptide, and insulin [7], γ -cells produce pancreatic polypeptide (PP) [8], δ -cells produce somatostatin [7], and ε -cells produce ghrelin [9]. Two of the pancreatic hormones play an essential role in the regulation of the blood glucose levels are insulin, which acts to lower it, and glucagon, which acts to raise it [10]. The balanced antagonistic action between them, maintain the glucose concentrations within the narrow range of 4–6 mM (70 to 110 mg/dL) [6]. However, both hormones are inhibited by somatostatin [11]. Production and secretion of the hormones by pancreatic cells are stimulated by external signals such as nutrients intake, fasting, or stress. Blood glucose levels decrease during periods of rest such as sleep, between meals, or during fasting periods. In these cases, pancreatic α -cells release glucagon to drive glycogenolysis and gluconeogenesis processes. Unlike, in postprandial state, i.e., after a meal ingestion, insulin is released from β -cells in the pancreas to reduce blood glucose levels via glycogenesis [12–14]. Insulin is released on demand but is produced and stored in large, dense-core vesicles that are recruited near the plasma membrane into the β -cells in the islets of Langerhans after stimulation so that insulin is readily available to upcoming stimuli [15]. Glucose is the main signal to release insulin from the pancreas, but free fatty acids and amino acids can increase glucose-induced insulin secretion through the so-called incretin effect. As before mentioned, the incretin effect is originated in the intestinal tract (mainly duodenum) once the food is ingested.

Insulin is a protein made up of 51 amino acids and when produced, it is first synthesized as a single polypeptide known as preproinsulin. Preproinsulin is an insulin gene encoded in 110 amino acids that are then processed into proinsulin. Proinsulin undergoes maturation into active insulin through the action of two different types of cells. One of them cleaves at 2 positions, releasing insulin and a fragment known as C-peptide [16], in an equimolar ratio, into the bloodstream.

Insulin is released from β-cells in the pancreas in two phases, first one is triggered in response to glucose levels and second one is triggered independently of sugar. Glucose and insulin in the bloodstream work together to avoid glucose from going out of range. Thus, Glucose is removed from the circulation thanks to the ability of insulin to cause insulin-dependent tissues to take up glucose [17–19]. Additionally, insulin promotes lipogenesis [20, 21], and the incorporation of amino acids into proteins [22] when it is in high concentrations. Different at low concentrations, which produce lipolysis in adipocytes, releasing free fatty acids by stimulating the use of lipids over glucose to satisfy energy needs at rest [23]. The release of insulin from β-cells is tightly regulated and exactly satisfies the metabolic demand for caloric nutrients in the body [16, 23]. Regarding C-peptide, it has been important to follow some insulin states that are difficult to measure [24].

4.2 Liver

The liver is perhaps considered the main blood glucose regulating organ in the human body because it functions in two different ways: controlling the rate of glucose absorption from the portal system and producing glucose from non-carbohydrate precursors or glycogen. As a curious fact, the liver is the only organ being irrigated by venous and arterial blood simultaneously. Venous irrigation comes from the portal system, provides the 75% of the blood supply, and carries blood rich in nutrients that were absorbed from the small intestine through enterocytes and hormones that were released by the pancreas. On the other hand, 25% of the remaining hepatic blood supply is arterial supply and is oxygen-rich blood coming from the aorta [4]. Blood from terminal branches of the hepatic artery and portal vein at the periphery of lobules is emptied into low-pressure vascular channels called sinusoids. Sinusoids are lined with endothelial cells and flanked circumferentially by plates of parenchymal cells-hepatocytes allowing the exchange of nutrients and oxygen between the blood and the hepatic cells [25]. Millions of sinusoids made up the lobules in the liver. Hepatocytes take up nutrients from blood in the sinusoid and once carry on all metabolic functions, return the substances resulting from the biochemical reactions to the blood via hepatic vein.

As mentioned earlier, the liver is a key organ in maintaining glucose concentrations in the desired range over both post-absorptive and postprandial states[1]. In the liver, four biochemical processes regarding glucose metabolism take place: glucose production from glycogen (glycogenolysis) and from non-carbohydrate precursors (gluconeogenesis), glucose consumption during the postprandial state (glucolysis), and glucose storage from the formation of glycogen (glycogenesis). Glucose phosphorylation (formation of glycogen) and dephosphorylation (formation of glucose from glycogen) occurs through the action of insulin and glucagon, respectively. Hepatocytes express dozens of enzymes that alternately turn on and off depending on whether blood glucose levels are rising or falling outside the normal range [26]. In the post-absorptive state, the human body is under fasting and the body must rely initially on stored glycogen to supply with glucose to the central nervous system and simultaneously regulate plasma glucose concentrations. If the fast is prolonged, the glycogen stores end, and the glucose dosage in the liver depends only on gluconeogenesis. On the other hand, after an ingested meal, i.e., in the postprandial state, absorbed nutrients enter the liver first from hepatic portal vein. Consequently, glycogen concentrations in the hepatocytes are restored by taking up a portion of the ingested glucose, minimizing the fluctuations of glycemia. In this case, gluconeogenesis is also occurring at a constant rate but the glucose output generated from glycogenolysis is suppressed. These result in a net switch from hepatic glucose output to hepatic glucose uptake [27].

Hepatic gluconeogenesis occurs by the action of additional groups of enzymes that are activated to start synthesizing glucose out of such precursors as amino acids and non-hexose carbohydrates such as glutamine, alanine, lactate and glycerol. Otherwise, the suppression of the glycogenolysis during the post-absorptive period and the activation of the glycogen synthesis during the postprandial period are mainly driven by stimulation of insulin secretion and suppression of glucagon secretion.

---

[1] Postprandial state is the time frame after a meal or food intake. Postabsorptive state is the period following absorption of nutrients from the digestive tract, that is, is the time when enterocytes stop providing nutrients to the hepatic portal circulation. Fasting is the willing abstinence or reduction from some or all food, drink, or both, for a long period of time (~ 8 hours).

In addition to being the primary site of glucose utilization during the postprandial period and glucose dosing during the post-absorption period, the liver is the primary site of clearance of insulin in the human body [28, 29]. Although the kidneys are the main site of extrasplanchnic insulin clearance, with additional contributions resulting from uptake and degradation by peripheral insulin-sensitive tissues, i.e., skeletal muscle and adipose tissue, the liver is the main organ responsible for clearance of exogenous and in particular endogenous insulin [30]. Insulin clearance from the liver is a dynamic process that can be modified within a few days under conditions of changing energy and, in particular, carbohydrate intake and before major changes in basal insulin secretion [31]. However, during first-pass transit near to 50% of the portal insulin is removed in the liver [32]. Removal of insulin from circulation does not imply the immediate destruction of the hormone [33]. A significant amount of receptor-bound insulin is released from the cell and reenters the circulation [34].

Hepatic glucose uptake is maximally stimulated by conditions that mimic the postprandial state, such as portal venous hyperglycemia and hyperinsulinemia [35]. Once glucose reaches the hepatocytes, it is phosphorylated to glucose 6-phosphate to synthesize glycogen, among other metabolic pathways. The ability of the liver to store glycogen is limited, and when glycogen concentrations reach maximum capacity, the hepatocytes initiate a process known as lipogenesis. Lipogenesis is the synthesis of excess glucose into fatty acids [36].

In conclusion, during short periods of fasting, glycogenolysis is the predominant source of glucose released into the bloodstream. However, during prolonged periods of fasting, the glycogen store is gradually depleted and glycogenolysis decreases as glycogen stores are depleted. So, gluconeogenesis becomes the predominant source of glucose for the human body. This unique ability of the human liver to store and release glucose is crucial to supporting periods of fasting.

4.3 Kidneys

The kidneys are two bean-shaped organs that are primarily engaged in filtering the blood and excreting waste. Filtration is about cleaning the blood to send it back into circulation, maintaining an overall fluid balance, creating hormones that help make red blood cells, promoting bone health, and regulating blood pressure [37]. Recent studies have demonstrated that kidneys also play a central role in glucose homeostasis through utilization of glucose, glucose production, and glucose filtration and reabsorption via sodium glucose co-transporters (SGLTs) and glucose transporters (GLUT-2). Moreover, the kidneys are an important site of insulin clearance from the systemic circulation, removing approximately 50% of peripheral insulin [34].

The kidneys have a super-specialized microscopic structural and functional unit called the nephron. Nephrons have the ability to distribute all functions in each of their parts. For example, the glomerulus is a network of small blood vessels known as capillaries located within Bowman's capsule. Blood is filtered across the glomerular capillaries into Bowman's space. These capillaries are multiple branches of the afferent arteriole but then converge at the efferent arteriole to exit the glomerulus and surround the renal tubules, including the proximal convoluted tubule, the proximal rectus tubule, the loop of Henle, the distal convoluted tubule, and the collecting ducts. Urine continually forms within the tubules to be excreted with waste products. Reabsorption, secretion, chemical reactions, and excretion also occur within the renal tubules [5].

The release of glucose occurs predominantly in the renal cortex, while the utilization of glucose is limited to the renal medulla. For this reason, the kidneys can be considered as two separate organs [38–42]. The renal medulla has an appreciable glucose phosphorylation capacity and, therefore, the ability to accumulate glycogen [42]. However, the kidney medulla consumes glucose anaerobically due to its low oxygen tension and low levels of oxidative enzymes, limiting the ability to produce glucose from glycogen. Consequently, lactate is the main metabolic end product of glucose taken up at the renal medulla, unlike carbon dioxide (CO_2) and water that are the end products of glucose uptake of aerobic energy requirements. In contrast, the renal cortex does not have appreciable glycogen stores [43] because has little glucose phosphorylation capacity but has a high level of oxidative enzymes like 6-phosphatase. Consequently, this part of the kidney does not take up and use much glucose, with oxidation of free fatty acids acting as the main source of energy [44]. Therefore, it is likely that glucose release by the normal kidney is primarily due to gluconeogenesis, that is, the synthesis of glucose-6-phosphate from non-carbohydrate precursors such as glutamine, lactate, alanine, glycerol, etc. [45], being glutamine the substrate with more specificity in the kidney but lactate the most abundant.

In addition, to its function both in the use and in the production of glucose, the kidneys contribute to the regulation of glucose in the blood by filtering and reabsorbing glucose. The glomeruli filter glucose once it reaches the kidneys, with other substances such as precursors and insulin, into the proximal tubules, where all the glucose is reabsorbed through the glucose transporting proteins present in the cell membranes within the proximal tubules [46], rendering the urine virtually glucose free. Before being reabsorbed, gluconeogenesis and glucose uptake occur. Glucose production is suppressed by insulin [45] or stimulated by non-carbohydrate precursors [41, 47]. An interesting fact is that GLUT-2 glucose transporters are independent of insulin and for that reason, the kidneys can continue their physiological functions even in states of insulin deficiency [23].

As before mentioned, gluconeogenesis in the human body is mainly carried out by the liver and the kidneys. In the post-absorptive state, both liver and kidneys release glucose into the circulation in comparable amounts [48]. However, in the postprandial state, although overall endogenous glucose release decreases substantially, renal gluconeogenesis increases by approximately twice liver gluconeogenesis. In this sense, the hepatic and renal glucose release into the circulation in the post-absorptive state correspond to the 25–30% and 20–25% of total glucose, respectively, while in postprandial state, hepatic gluconeogenesis is reduced by $\sim$ 80% and the release of glucose molecules generated via this pathway decreases as these molecules are largely directed into the formation of hepatic glycogen. As a consequence of these changes, renal gluconeogenesis increases accounts for $\sim$ 60% of postprandial endogenous glucose release [49].

4.4 Gastrointestinal tract

The gastrointestinal (GI) tract is an organ system, consisting of the mouth, esophagus, stomach, and intestines, where humans ingest food, digest it to extract and absorb energy and nutrients, and expel the remaining waste as feces. However, the literature on glucose homeostasis includes the gastrointestinal tract as a complete organ without taking into account the physiological functions and glucose consumption of the stomach and small intestine as separate organs involved in glucose metabolism.

Meal is ingested through mouth and enters in the stomach to be mixed. The rate at which nutrients pass from the stomach to the duodenum, i.e., crossing the pyloric valve, is known as the gastric emptying rate and is a key determinant of postprandial glucose flow. In the fed state, glucose homeostasis becomes more complex as the gastrointestinal tract becomes a second source of exogenous glucose. Marked and rapid changes in glucose flux occur as a result of the considerable inflow of meal-derived glucose into the circulation [50]. The delivery of nutrients from the gastrointestinal tract occurs through an important rate limiting mechanical step in the form of gastric emptying rate: the rate at which the pylorus allows small boluses of gastric content to pass into the duodenum for downstream absorption. Importantly, neither insulin nor glucagon has direct effects on gastric emptying and exogenous glucose diffusion from the gastrointestinal tract [51]. However, the influx of glucose is accompanied by secretion of several other regulatory hormones of glucose including amylin from β -cells in the pancreas and glucose-dependent inhibitory peptide (GIP), glucagon-like peptide-1 (GLP-1), and cholecystokinin (CCK) from endocrine cells in the small intestine. Endocrine cells in the small intestine collectively influence glucose homeostasis via several mechanisms of action including regulation of insulin and glucagon responses, as well as the modulation of nutrient passage from the gastrointestinal tract to appropriate tissue stores [52–54].

A key contribution of the GI tract on glucose homeostasis is the incretin effect. This physiological response came from the observation that an oral glucose load results in an increased insulin response compared to the response seen when intravenous glucose administration replicates the same changes in plasma glucose [55, 56]. In other words, when glucose is ingested orally, an augmented β -cell response is observed as a result of a signal passed from the gut. The two hormones responsible for this effect are GIP and GLP-1. Both GIP, secreted from enteroendocrine K-cells in the proximal small bowel, and GLP-1, secreted from enteroendocrine L-cells in the distal ileum and colon, have a strong insulinotropic effect [57]. Additionally, GLP-1 inhibits postprandial glucagon secretion in a glucose-dependent manner, slows gastric emptying, and reduces food intake, contributing to postprandial glucose regulation [58]. Regarding the role of the stomach in the metabolism of glucose, the stomach must consume glucose to generate the energy necessary to mechanically carry out the digestion process. Although the consumption of glucose in the stomach is relatively low, it can affect the concentration of glucose in the bloodstream.

4.5 Brain

The human brain depends on glucose as its main source of energy; neurons have the highest energy demand [59] of all types of cells in the human body, requiring continuous delivery of glucose from blood. Glucose metabolism provides the fuel for physiological brain function through the generation of ATP, the foundation for neuronal and non-neuronal cellular maintenance, as well as the generation of neurotransmittersTherefore, tight regulation of glucose metabolism is critical to brain physiology. In this sense, the alteration of glucose metabolism in the brain is the basis of several diseases that affect both the brain and the entire organism. Glucose is required in the brain to provide the precursors of neurotransmitter synthesis and ATP to fuel their actions. Additionally, glucose is important for the brain's energy demands unrelated to signaling. Cellular compartmentalization of glucose transport and metabolism are closely related to local regulation of blood flow, and glucose-sensing neurons govern the brain–body nutrient axis. Glucose metabolism is connected to cell death pathways by the glucose-metabolizing enzymes [60]. Thus, disruption glucose delivery pathways and metabolism leads to debilitating brain diseases.

The brain uses about 120 g of glucose per day - 60-70% of the body's total glucose metabolism. The brain has little stored glucose and has no additional sources of stored energy. Brain function begins to become seriously affected when glucose levels fall below $\sim 40\, mg\,/\,dL$. Glucose levels significantly below this can lead to permanent damage and death. The brain cannot use fatty acids for energy (fatty acids do not cross the blood–brain barrier of the neurons), but ketone bodies can enter the brain and be used for energy in hypoglycemic conditions. In this sense, the brain can only use glucose, or, under conditions of starvation, ketone bodies (acetoacetate and hydroxybutyrate) for energy.

5. Conclusions

Glucose, as the main source of energy for the cells of the human body, is regulated by the joint work of several organs. Each organ involved in this glucose regulatory mechanism plays an important role that cannot be disregarded. Metabolic disorders such as diabetes mellitus are supposed to only cause an alteration of the pancreas, but recent studies indicate that when a condition such as diabetes mellitus appears, the rest of the organs are also significantly affected. For this reason, it is important to have a healthy lifestyle both to prevent diseases that cause metabolic disorders if you do not have them or to have better control of blood glucose levels and prevent possible complications that these disorders can cause.

Author details

Laura Lema-Pérez
National University of Colombia, Medellín, Colombia

*Address all correspondence to: llemap@unal.edu.co

References

[1] F. E. T. Al, C. S. Fink, P. Hamosh, and M. Hamosh, "Fat Digestion in the Stomach: Stability of Lingual Lipase in the Gastric Environment," no. 62, 1984.

[2] K. S. Saladin, *Anatomy & Physiology: The Unity of Form and Function*, 7th Edició. McGraw-Hill Education, 2014.

[3] L. Poretsky, *Principles of Diabetes*, 2nd ed., vol. 53, no. 9. Springer, Boston, MA, 2009.

[4] J. A. Fernandez-Tresguerres *et al.*, *Fisiología humana*, 3rd ed. 2005.

[5] John E. Hall PhD, *Textbook of Medical Physiology*, 13th ed. Guyton Physiology, 2015.

[6] P. V. Röder, B. Wu, Y. Liu, and W. Han, "Pancreatic regulation of glucose homeostasis," *Exp. Mol. Med.*, vol. 48, no. November 2015, p. e219, 2016, doi: 10.1038/emm.2016.6.

[7] M. Brissova *et al.*, "Assessment of human pancreatic islet architecture and composition by laser scanning confocal microscopy.," *J. Histochem. Cytochem. Off. J. Histochem. Soc.*, vol. 53, no. 9, pp. 1087-1097, Sep. 2005, doi: 10.1369/jhc.5C6684.2005.

[8] G. Katsuura, A. Asakawa, and A. Inui, "Roles of pancreatic polypeptide in regulation of food intake," *Peptides*, vol. 23, no. 2, pp. 323-329, 2002, doi: https://doi.org/10.1016/S0196-9781(01)00604-0.

[9] N. Wierup, H. Svensson, H. Mulder, and F. Sundler, "The ghrelin cell: a novel developmentally regulated islet cell in the human pancreas.," *Regul. Pept.*, vol. 107, no. 1-3, pp. 63-69, Jul. 2002, doi: 10.1016/s0167-0115(02)00067-8.

[10] B. Göke, "Islet cell function: α and β cells - Partners towards normoglycaemia," *Int. J. Clin. Pract. Suppl.*, vol. 159, pp. 2-7, 2008, doi: 10.1111/j.1742-1241.2007.01686.x.

[11] A. C. Hauge-Evans *et al.*, "Somatostatin secreted by islet delta-cells fulfills multiple roles as a paracrine regulator of islet function.," *Diabetes*, vol. 58, no. 2, pp. 403-11, 2009, doi: 10.2337/db08-0792.

[12] S. Y. Kim *et al.*, "SREBP-1c mediates the insulin-dependent hepatic glucokinase expression," *J. Biol. Chem.*, vol. 279, no. 29, pp. 30823-30829, 2004, doi: 10.1074/jbc.M313223200.

[13] T. B. Miller and J. Larner, "Mechanism of control of hepatic glycogenesis by insulin," *J. Biol. Chem.*, vol. 248, no. 10, pp. 3483-3488, 1973.

[14] N. A. Syed and R. L. Khandelwal, "Reciprocal regulation of glycogen phosphorylase and glycogen synthase by insulin involving phosphatidylinositol-3 kinase and protein phosphatase-1 in HepG2 cells.," *Mol. Cell. Biochem.*, vol. 211, no. 1-2, pp. 123-136, Aug. 2000, doi: 10.1023/a:1007159422667.

[15] M. Hao, X. Li, M. A. Rizzo, J. V Rocheleau, B. M. Dawant, and D. W. Piston, "Regulation of two insulin granule populations within the reserve pool by distinct calcium sources," *J. Cell Sci.*, vol. 118, no. 24, pp. 5873-5884, 2005, doi: 10.1242/jcs.02684.

[16] Z. Fu, E. R. Gilbert, and D. Liu, "Regulation of Insulin Synthesis and Secretion and Pancreatic Beta-Cell Dysfunction in Diabetes," *Curr. Diabetes Rev.*, vol. 9, no. 1, pp. 25-53, 2013, doi: 10.2174/157339913804143225.

[17] A. H. Khan and J. E. Pessin, "Insulin regulation of glucose uptake: a complex interplay of intracellular signalling pathways.," *Diabetologia*, vol. 45, no. 11,

pp. 1475-1483, Nov. 2002, doi: 10.1007/s00125-002-0974-7.

[18] A. D. Kohn, S. A. Summers, M. J. Birnbaum, and R. A. Roth, "Expression of a constitutively active Akt Ser/Thr kinase in 3T3-L1 adipocytes stimulates glucose uptake and glucose transporter 4 translocation," *J. Biol. Chem.*, vol. 271, no. 49, pp. 31372-31378, 1996, doi: 10.1074/jbc.271.49.31372.

[19] A. Zisman *et al.*, "Targeted disruption of the glucose transporter 4 selectively in muscle causes insulin resistance and glucose intolerance," *Nat. Med.*, vol. 6, no. 8, pp. 924-928, 2000, doi: 10.1038/78693.

[20] P. G. McTernan *et al.*, "Insulin and rosiglitazone regulation of lipolysis and lipogenesis in human adipose tissue in vitro.," *Diabetes*, vol. 51, no. 5, pp. 1493-1498, May 2002, doi: 10.2337/diabetes.51.5.1493.

[21] P. E. Walton and T. D. Etherton, "Stimulation of lipogenesis by insulin in swine adipose tissue: antagonism by porcine growth hormone.," *J. Anim. Sci.*, vol. 62, no. 6, pp. 1584-1595, Jun. 1986, doi: 10.2527/jas1986.6261584x.

[22] G. Biolo, R. Y. Declan Fleming, and R. R. Wolfe, "Physiologic hyperinsulinemia stimulates protein synthesis and enhances transport of selected amino acids in human skeletal muscle.," *J. Clin. Invest.*, vol. 95, no. 2, pp. 811-819, Feb. 1995, doi: 10.1172/JCI117731.

[23] E. Mann and M. D. Bellin, "Secretion of Insulin in Response to Diet and Hormones," *Pancreapedia*, no. 1, 2016, doi: 10.3998/panc.2016.3.

[24] E. Leighton, C. A. Sainsbury, and G. C. Jones, "A Practical Review of C-Peptide Testing in Diabetes," *Diabetes Ther.*, vol. 8, no. 3, pp. 475-487, 2017, doi: 10.1007/s13300-017-0265-4.

[25] E. Chalhoub, "an in Silico Liver : Model of Gluconeogensis," *PhD thesis*, no. March, 2013.

[26] C. Postic, R. Dentin, and J. Girard, "Role of the liver in the control of carbohydrate and lipid homeostasis," *Diabetes Metab.*, vol. 30, no. 5, pp. 398-408, 2004, doi: 10.1016/S1262-3636(07)70133-7.

[27] A. D. C. Mary Courtney Moore, Katie C. Coate, Jason J. Winnick, Zhibo An, "Regulation of hepatic glucose uptake and storage in vivo.," *Adv. Nutr.*, vol. 3, no. 3, pp. 286-294, 2012, doi: 10.3945/an.112.002089.

[28] W. C. Duckworth, F. G. Hamel, and D. E. Peavy, "Hepatic metabolism of insulin," *Am. J. Med.*, vol. 85, no. 5, Supplement 1, pp. 71-76, 1988, doi: https://doi.org/10.1016/0002-9343(88)90399-3.

[29] H. Sato, T. Terasaki, H. Mizuguchi, K. Okumura, and A. Tsuji, "Receptor-recycling model of clearance and distribution of insulin in the perfused mouse liver," *Diabetologia*, vol. 34, no. 9, pp. 613-621, 1991, doi: 10.1007/BF00400989.

[30] E. Ferrannini, J. Wahren, O. K. Faber, P. Felig, C. Binder, and R. A. DeFronzo, "Splanchnic and renal metabolism of insulin in human subjects: a dose-response study," *Am. J. Physiol. Metab.*, vol. 244, no. 6, pp. E517–E527, Jun. 1983, doi: 10.1152/ajpendo.1983.244.6.E517.

[31] K. N. Bojsen-Møller, A. M. Lundsgaard, S. Madsbad, B. Kiens, and J. J. Holst, "Hepatic insulin clearance in regulation of systemic insulin concentrations-role of carbohydrate and energy availability," *Diabetes*, vol. 67, no. 11, pp. 2129-2136, 2018, doi: 10.2337/db18-0539.

[32] M. M. I. Hennes, A. Dua, and A. H. Kissebah, "Effects of Free Fatty Acids

and Glucose on Splanchnic Insulin Dynamics," *Diabetes*, vol. 46, no. 1, pp. 57-62, 1997, doi: 10.2337/diab.46.1.57.

[33] X. Y. Ma *et al.*, "Preliminary study of oral polylactide microcapsulated insulin in vitro and in vivo.," *Diabetes. Obes. Metab.*, vol. 2, no. 4, pp. 243-250, Aug. 2000, doi: 10.1046/j.1463-1326.2000.00080.x.

[34] W. C. Duckworth, R. G. Bennett, and F. G. Hamel, "Insulin Degradation: Progress and Potential*," *Endocr. Rev.*, vol. 19, no. 5, pp. 608-624, 1998, doi: 10.1210/edrv.19.5.0349.

[35] M. J. Pagliassotti and A. D. Cherrington, "Regulation of net hepatic glucose uptake in vivo.," *Annu. Rev. Physiol.*, vol. 54, pp. 847-860, 1992, doi: 10.1146/annurev.ph.54.030192.004215.

[36] M. M. Adeva-Andany, N. Pérez-Felpete, C. Fernández-Fernández, C. Donapetry-García, and C. Pazos-García, "Liver glucose metabolism in humans," *Biosci. Rep.*, vol. 36, no. 6, pp. 1-15, 2016, doi: 10.1042/BSR20160385.

[37] I. Sgouralis and A. T. Layton, "HHS Public Access," *Math. Biosci.*, vol. 264, pp. 8-20, 2015, doi: 10.1016/j.mbs.2015.02.016.

[38] A. C. Schoolwerth, B. C. Smith, and R. M. Culpepper, "Renal gluconeogenesis.," *Miner. Electrolyte Metab.*, vol. 14, no. 6, pp. 347-361, 1988.

[39] H. J. Adrogué, "Glucose homeostasis and the kidney," *Kidney Int.*, vol. 42, no. 5, pp. 1266-1282, 1992, doi: 10.1038/ki.1992.414.

[40] W. G. Guder and B. D. Ross, "Enzyme distribution along the nephron," *Kidney Int.*, vol. 26, no. 2, pp. 101-111, 1984, doi: 10.1038/ki.1984.143.

[41] C. L. Triplitt, "Understanding the kidneys' role in blood glucose regulation," *Am J Manag Care*, vol. 18, no. 1 Suppl, pp. S11-6, 2012.

[42] G. Wirthensohn and W. G. Guder, "Renal Substrate Metabolism," *Physiol. Rev.*, vol. 66, no. 2, pp. 469-497, 1986, [Online]. Available: http://www.ncbi.nlm.nih.gov/pubmed/10909977.

[43] C. Biava, A. Grossman, and M. West, "Ultrastructural observations on renal glycogen in normal and pathologic human kidneys.," *Lab. Invest.*, vol. 15, no. 1 Pt 2, pp. 330-356, Jan. 1966.

[44] J. E. Gerich, "Role of the kidney in normal glucose homeostasis and in the hyperglycaemia of diabetes mellitus : therapeutic implications," *DIABETICMedicine*, vol. 27, no. i, pp. 136-142, 2010, doi: 10.1111/j.1464-5491.2009.02894.x.

[45] M. Stumvoll, C. Meyer, A. Mitrakou, V. Nadkarni, and J. E. Gerich, "Renal glucose production and utilization : new aspects in humans," *Diabetologia*, vol. 40, pp. 749-757, 1997.

[46] O. Marsenic, "Glucose Control by the Kidney: An Emerging Target in Diabetes," *Am. J. Kidney Dis.*, vol. 53, no. 5, pp. 875-883, May 2009, doi: 10.1053/j.ajkd.2008.12.031.

[47] M. Alsahli and J. E. Gerich, "Renal glucose metabolism in normal physiological conditions and in diabetes," *Diabetes Res. Clin. Pract.*, vol. 33, pp. 1-9, 2017, doi: 10.1016/j.diabres.2017.07.033.

[48] M. Stumvoll, U. Chintalapudi, G. Perriello, S. Welle, O. Gutierrez, and J. Gerich, "Uptake and release of glucose by the human kidney. Postabsorptive rates and responses to epinephrine.," *J. Clin. Invest.*, vol. 96, no. 5, pp. 2528-2533, Nov. 1995, doi: 10.1172/JCI118314.

[49] C. Meyer *et al.*, "Role of human liver , kidney , and skeletal muscle in postprandial glucose homeostasis," *Am*

J Physiol Endocrinol Metab, vol. 282, pp. 419-427, 2002.

[50] G. Pehling, P. Tessari, J. E. Gerich, M. W. Haymond, F. J. Service, and R. A. Rizza, "Abnormal meal carbohydrate disposition in insulin-dependent diabetes. Relative contributions of endogenous glucose production and initial splanchnic uptake and effect of intensive insulin therapy," *J. Clin. Invest.*, vol. 74, no. 3, pp. 985-991, 1984, doi: 10.1172/JCI111519.

[51] G. Jiang and B. B. Zhang, "Glucagon and regulation of glucose metabolism," *Am. J. Physiol. Metab.*, vol. 284, no. 4, pp. E671–E678, 2003, doi: 10.1152/ajpendo.00492.2002.

[52] J. J. Holst, "Glucagon-like Peptide 1 (GLP-1): An Intestinal Hormone, Signalling Nutritional Abundance, with an Unusual Therapeutic Potential.," *Trends Endocrinol. Metab.*, vol. 10, no. 6, pp. 229-235, Aug. 1999, doi: 10.1016/s1043-2760(99)00157-5.

[53] J. J. Meier, M. A. Nauck, W. E. Schmidt, and B. Gallwitz, "Gastric Inhibitory Polypeptide: the neglected incretin revisited," *Regul. Pept.*, vol. 107, no. 1, pp. 1-13, 2002, doi: https://doi.org/10.1016/S0167-0115(02)00039-3.

[54] G. Sachs, N. Zeng, and C. Prinz, "PHYSIOLOGY OF ISOLATED GASTRIC ENDOCRINE CELLS," *Annu. Rev. Physiol.*, vol. 59, no. 1, pp. 243-256, Oct. 1997, doi: 10.1146/annurev.physiol.59.1.243.

[55] M. A. Nauck *et al.*, "Incretin effects of increasing glucose loads in man calculated from venous insulin and C-peptide responses.," *J. Clin. Endocrinol. Metab.*, vol. 63, no. 2, pp. 492-498, Aug. 1986, doi: 10.1210/jcem-63-2-492.

[56] M. J. Perley and D. M. Kipnis, "Plasma insulin responses to oral and intravenous glucose: studies in normal and diabetic sujbjects.," *J. Clin. Invest.*, vol. 46, no. 12, pp. 1954-1962, Dec. 1967, doi: 10.1172/JCI105685.

[57] D. J. Drucker and M. A. Nauck, "The incretin system: glucagon-like peptide-1 receptor agonists and dipeptidyl peptidase-4 inhibitors in type 2 diabetes.," *Lancet (London, England)*, vol. 368, no. 9548, pp. 1696-1705, Nov. 2006, doi: 10.1016/S0140-6736(06)69705-5.

[58] J. J. Holst and J. Gromada, "Role of incretin hormones in the regulation of insulin secretion in diabetic and nondiabetic humans.," *Am. J. Physiol. Endocrinol. Metab.*, vol. 287, no. 2, pp. E199-206, Aug. 2004, doi: 10.1152/ajpendo.00545.2003.

[59] C. Howarth, P. Gleeson, and D. Attwell, "Updated energy budgets for neural computation in the neocortex and cerebellum," *J. Cereb. Blood Flow Metab.*, vol. 32, no. 7, pp. 1222-1232, 2012, doi: 10.1038/jcbfm.2012.35.

[60] P. Mergenthaler, U. Lindauer, G. A. Dienel, and A. Meisel, "Sugar for the brain: the role of glucose in physiological and pathological brain function," *Trends Neurosci.*, vol. 36, no. 10, pp. 587-597, 2014, doi: 10.1016/j.tins.2013.07.001.Sugar.

Chapter 9

Application of a Pedometer for the Management of Impaired Glucose Tolerance in Pregnant Women

Mariko Ueno, Mitsue Muraoka and Koichiro Takagi

Abstract

The proper management of impaired glucose tolerance (IGT) in pregnant women is important for both obstetricians and diabetologists as this condition is of interest to both obstetrics and internal medicine. Although nutritional intervention along with insulin treatment is the mainstream approach of IGT treatment in pregnant women, exercise intervention is another important component of the IGT management. A pedometer is a useful tool for objective exercise evaluation. Nonetheless, its application in the management of IGT in pregnant women is limited. On the other hand, with the widespread use of smartphones equipped with pedometer function, exercise by walking is easily monitored and utilised in both healthy pregnant women and pregnant women with obesity and impaired glucose tolerance. In this chapter, we review the present perspective on the use of a pedometer in the management of IGT in pregnant women by introducing our recently published work.

Keywords: pregnancy, impaired glucose tolerance, gestational diabetes mellitus, exercise, pedometer

1. Introduction

Followed by recent substantial progress in the field of IT, smartphones equipped with a pedometer function have enabled us to measure the amount of steps we take daily and to estimate a daily caloric expenditure, which are useful tools of health self-monitoring. Pedometer or pedometer-equipped smartphones might theoretically help improving health of the people with conditions such as obesity, locomotive problems, and impaired glucose tolerance. Nonetheless, there are a few reports demonstrating the effectiveness of a pedometer in weight control and metabolic control in non-pregnant individuals as well as in pregnant women partly because the difficulties in the setting of quantitative outcome of the study or the special nature of the subjects those who are reluctant to exercise. The management of impaired glucose tolerance requires strict blood glucose control through a proper management of diet and exercise. However, the difficulty in quantification of the amount of exercise may let obstetricians and internists to prefer too strict nutritional control or easier use of insulin. We believe that exercise quantification, which is an important part of glycemic control, might be beneficial for the management of impaired glucose tolerance. In this chapter, we review a recent report on the role of a pedometer during effective management of impaired glucose tolerance during pregnancy.

IntechOpen

2. Maternal weight gain during pregnancy

Women gain approximately 12.5 kg of body weight during pregnancy [1]. This increase is due to the uterus and its contents, i.e., the foetus, the placenta, and the amniotic fluid, but also due to enlarged breasts with the extracellular fluid. This compartmentalisation makes the assessment of obesity and weight gain difficult during a short period of pregnancy, which lasts 9 months. Weight gain during pregnancy is associated with offspring obesity and cardiometabolic traits in early childhood in a trimester-specific fashion [2]. Greater rate of gestational weight gain in the first trimester of pregnancy was associated with increased risk of overweight and obesity from 2 years to 4 years of age, high waist circumference, high sum of skinfold thickness and higher diastolic blood pressure at 4 years of age. In contrast, Greater rate of gestational weight gain during the second and the third trimesters was associated with greater risk of large-for-gestational age neonates [2]. Our group has recently reported that in hyperemesis gravidarum, in which maternal undernutrition occurs in the first trimester of pregnancy, the pattern of foetal head growth differs from that of the normal pregnancy [3]. Moreover, the weight gain in slim and obese women should not be the same because of the differences in their nutritional demands during pregnancy. Association of gestational weight gain with adverse maternal and infant outcomes has been demonstrated by the LifeCycle Project-Maternal Obesity and Childhood Outcomes Study Group [4]. From this large scale meta-analysis of 25 cohort studies, they concluded that maternal prepregnancy BMI, and to a lesser extent gestational weight gain, are associated with risks of adverse maternal and infant adverse outcomes. Gestational weight gain ranges that were associated with lower risks for adverse outcomes were 14.0 Kg to less than 16.0 Kg for underweight women, 10.0 Kg to less than 18.0 Kg for normal weight women, 2.0 Kg to less than 16.0 Kg for overweight women, and 2.0 Kg or less than 6.0 Kg for grade I obese women [4]. The Institute of Medicine and National Research Council revised its guidelines for weight gain during pregnancy according to the prepregnant nutritional status estimated by the pre-pregnancy BMI [5]. In Japan, according to the Healthy Parents and Children 21 by the Health, Labour and Welfare of Japan Government, the weight gain guidelines are 10–12 Kg for women with a pre-pregnancy BMI less than 18.5 Kg/m^2, 7–12 Kg for women with a pre-pregnancy BMI of 18.5 to 25 Kg/m^2, and appropriate increase for those with prepregnant BMI over 25 Kg/m^2 [6]. However, adherence to the gestational weight gain recommendations seems to be limited for obese women in preventing increased birth weights [7]. In addition, behavioural interventions by the healthcare providers for the obese women are practically complicated due to several factors such as educational levels, ethnicity, and socio-economical levels. In particular, weight control is of huge importance during pregnancy complicated with diabetes and gestational diabetes, in which obesity is strongly associated with their pathophysiology.

3. Carbohydrate metabolism during pregnancy

The energy metabolism of women changes dramatically during pregnancy, as sufficient nutrition for the foetus must be provided. The foetus is nourished through the maternal-foetal interface called the placenta, by which essential nutrients, including the main foetal energy source—glucose and oxygen, are transported from the mother to the foetus. In line, foetal waste products such as carbon dioxide are transported from the foetus to the mother via the placenta. Various hormones are involved in the promotion of insulin resistance. Prolactin (PRL) and human placental lactogen (hPL) have been reported to suppress glucose uptake through the action of GLUT4 [8, 9]. Moreover, a study of the effect of oestradiol (E2) and progesterone (P4) on the action of insulin has shown that P4 suppresses insulin signalling and reduces glucose uptake through a step-wise process by reducing the amount of protein in the insulin receptor to suppress the transport of GLUT4 to cell membranes, downregulating the PI3-kinase-independent pathway [8, 9]. It has also been shown that insulin sensitivity is reduced through the suppression of tyrosine phosphorylation in insulin receptors via increased E2 blood levels that have been observed in the latter half of human pregnancy [8, 9].

4. Impaired glucose tolerance during pregnancy

As mentioned in the previous section, pregnancy itself is to some extent diabetogenic in its third trimester. Thus, women who are obese or relatively older when becoming pregnant may have a higher risk of developing glucose intolerance during pregnancy. This condition is known as gestational diabetes. Alternatively, a woman may have pregestational diabetes or undiagnosed diabetes until she becomes pregnant. In all of these cases, the foetus is over-nourished, which results in obesity in new-born babies with higher perinatal morbidity and mortality and a higher risk of developing diabetes in the near future in cases of gestational diabetes [9]. As mentioned previously, a special metabolic change of pregnancy let a pregnant women change into insulin-resistant condition. For this reason, the maximum insulin demand in the third trimester of pregnancy of prepregnant diabetic women with type I and type 2 diabetes mellitus are reported to be 1.5 times and 2 times higher than those of pre-pregnant demands, respectively [10]. The fundamental approach in the management of impaired glucose tolerance in pregnancy is to keep blood glucose levels as close to the non-pregnant levels as possible [11]. There are two important factors which need to be considered when achieving this goal, namely energy intake and energy expenditure. Measurements of blood glucose levels, glycosylated haemoglobin or albumin are routinely employed for the monitoring of diabetic control [12]. However, suitable energy expenditure, in other words, suitable exercise has not been studied in detail to date.

5. Exercise and carbohydrate metabolism during pregnancy

Regular exercise is recommended during pregnancy. In 2009, The American College of Obstetricians and Gynaecologists recommended that in the absence of contraindications such as pre-existing medical complications and pregnancy complications, pregnant women should be encouraged to engage in regular, moderate-intensity physical activity for 30 minutes or more daily [13]. Antenatal lifestyle interventions including exercise and diet for obese women also improved infant adiposity as well as maternal lifestyle behaviours at 6 months postpartum [14]. There are some evidence suggesting that pregnant women who engage in recreational physical activity have 50% lower risk of gestational diabetes and 40% risk reduction for preeclampsia [15].

Studies concerning the relationship between exercise and blood glucose levels have shown that, in healthy individuals, moderate amounts of exercise increase gluconeogenesis in the liver and other organs by decreasing insulin levels and elevating glucagon levels [8, 9]. Eighty percent of the glucose is used by skeletal muscles, making them the major user of carbohydrates in the body [9]. There are two pathways for the use of carbohydrates in the skeletal muscles. One is a pathway by which the GLUT4 that is present in muscle cells is transported to the surface of cell membranes (translocation) and glucose uptake then occurs when insulin binds with receptors on the surface of the muscle cell membranes [9]. The other pathway is one by which insulin-independent glucose uptake is made possible by translocation of GLUT4 by adenosine monophosphate-dependent protein kinase that is activated in conjunction with muscle contractions [9]. Although the GLUT4 on the cell surface disappears 2 to 3 hours after exercise, the turn-over of the translocation of GLUT4 is upregulated by the exercise in response to the same levels of blood insulin concentrations [9]. Furthermore, the gene transcription of GLUT4 is enhanced after 10 or more hours after exercise [9]. As a result, even though glucose from the blood is uptaken by skeletal muscles, blood glucose levels are almost unaltered. However, although patients with type 2 DM are able to increase the uptake of glucose into skeletal muscle through exercise, they experience a decrease in the blood glucose level through the suppression of gluconeogenesis in the liver due to hyperinsulinemia [9]. Further, post-exercise promotion of glycogen synthesis and insulin sensitivity causes a drop in blood glucose levels. Recently, participation of angiotensin-(1–7), a vasoactive peptide of the renin-angiotensin system is demonstrated in enhanced skeletal muscle insulin sensitivity after a bout of exercise [16]. It is known that patients treated with insulin and hypoglycaemic agents are particularly susceptible to hypoglycaemia from the day of exercise to the following day [8]. Similar to type 2 DM, carbohydrate metabolism switches into insulin resistance in the latter half of pregnancy. Therefore, one may speculate that the blood glucose levels might be influenced by exercise during pregnancy. However, Artal et al. measured the blood glucose levels, insulin concentrations, and glucagon concentrations in women in the third trimester of normal pregnancies before and after a 15-minute treadmill exercise. The results indicated that the post-exercise blood glucose level and insulin level did not change, but that the glucagon level was elevated [17]. In contrast, Soultanakis et al. showed that continuous prolonged exercise in pregnancy with about 55% VO_2 or higher could result in hypoglycaemia after 45–60 minutes of continuous exercise, suggesting the importance of appropriate exercise plans in the management of blood glucose levels in women with impaired glucose tolerance [18]. In line, Artal suggested that one moderate bout of exercise of 30–45 minutes/day and one bout of exercise after each meal to burn at least 200 kcal or more per day is effective in obtaining or maintaining euglycemia during pregnancy [17]. It is noteworthy that a regular programme of exercise before pregnancy appears to lower the risk of developing gestational diabetes mellitus (GDM) [19].

6. Application of a pedometer as an exercise-monitoring tool

A rationale for the application of a pedometer for exercise quantification has been tested in non-pregnant women using doubly-labelled water, a gold standard measurement of free-living energy expenditure with that of the accelerometer. The study demonstrated that the accelerometer is an alternative objective tool for the evaluation of exercise quantitatively in non-pregnant individuals [20]. Furthermore, Harrison et al. compared the accelerometer and pedometer as well as the subjective exercise assessment questionnaire, the International Physical Activity Questionnaire (IPAQ), showing that the pedometer was superior to the accelerometer and IPAQ in an objective assessment of exercise during pregnancy [21].

7. Application of a pedometer as a health care improving tool

7.1 Non-pregnant condition

The application of a pedometer for health improvement has been examined in the non-pregnancy context. Richardson et al. reported a meta-analysis of pedometer-based walking interventions and weight loss [22]. They searched 6 electronic databases and found nine studies which met their inclusion criteria. Those studies demonstrated that pedometer-based walking programs resulted in a modest amount of weight loss, on average 0.05 kg per week during the interventions. Mitsui et al. showed gender differences in the relationship between steps/day and BMI in Japanese adults [23]. Walker et al. showed that a 10,000 steps per day for 6 months resulted in a 3.0 cm loss in waist circumference, whereas there were no differences in body mass index among 142 subjects, including both genders [24]. The application of pedometer was examined for ovulation induction along with administration of clomiphene citrate in overweight women with polycystic ovary syndrome with greater number of spontaneous ovulation and pregnancy [25]. With respect to the effect of exercise monitored with a pedometer on carbohydrate metabolism, Huus et al. showed that physical activity assessed with a pedometer in healthy schoolchildren at the age of 8 and 12 longitudinally improved insulin sensitivity and decreased fasting C-peptide irrespective of the BMI [26]. This report is interesting because they investigated the association of exercise monitored with pedometer and insulin sensitivity qualitatively.

7.2 Pregnant condition

The clinical use of pedometers in obese pregnant women has been a controversial topic. Streuling et al. performed a meta-analysis on clinical trials which dealt with the application of a pedometer in the management of gestational weight gain [27]. Out of 1380 studies, they identified 12 trials that met their inclusion criteria. In seven trials, gestational weight gain was lower in the exercise group than in the control group, whereas five trials showed a lower GWG in the control groups. In Asia, Jiang et al. reported that pregnant women being physically active assessed by pedometer had less weight gain during pregnancy [28]. In this report, the activity levels were divided into 4 groups as sedentary (< 5000 daily steps), low active (5000–7000 daily steps), somewhat active (7500–10,000 daily steps) and active (≥10,000 daily steps). In accordance with Jiang's report, Cohen and Koski reported that both more than 5000 steps/day assessed by pedometer and daily energy intakes within 300 kcal of estimated energy requirements minimised postpartum weight retention of healthy pregnant women [29]. Although the application of a pedometer for the control of gestational weight gain seems controversial based on the abovementioned meta-analysis, one of the most important questions is related to the use of a pedometer by obese women, because they may be reluctant to exercise and that could be one of the reasons why they are obese. Even in a recent multi-institutional study conducted in Australia which used a randomised controlled trial in order to assess a pedometer-based intervention to increase activity and reduce excessive weight gain in pregnant women, the conclusion of the study showed negative results with the notion that the improvement of compliance with activity data recording and behavioural interventions delivered [30]. However, there are promising reports on the use of a pedometer for the management of overweight and obese pregnant women by active intervention with individualised nutritional support and individual exercise plans. For example, one study described an intervention at

16 to 20 weeks of gestation in overweight and obese women. The average number of steps after the intervention was over 10,000, along with the intake of 2000 kcal/day. This approach resulted in the prevention of excessive weight gain as well as excessive postpartum weight retention [31]. The study clearly demonstrated that both nutritional and exercise interventions are necessary in order to achieve reasonable outcomes in the management of glucose metabolism in obese pregnant women. In comparison of a smartphone pedometer with a reference pedometer, The Yamax Digiwalker, Tokyo, Japan, a smartphone pedometer is even superior at a low walking speed, suggesting a smartphone pedometer might be superior to pregnant women who are not expected to walk faster. [32]. So, there is no problem in using a smartphone pedometer instead of stand-alone pedometer.

8. Application of a pedometer for the management of impaired glucose tolerance in pregnant women

It is reasonable to assume that walking quantified by a pedometer is beneficial for the management of impaired glucose tolerance not only in non-pregnant subjects but also in pregnant subjects. Dahjio et al. reported a study on pedometer-monitored walking for the management of glucose in non-pregnant individuals. They examined a 12-week aerobic exercise training program monitored with a pedometer in type II diabetic Cameroonian women [33]. The subjects showed a significant reduction in body weight, waist circumference, and mean glycaemia after 12 weeks of the program. However, no study so far has reported the use of a pedometer in pregnant women with impaired glucose tolerance. Hence, we examined the feasibility of using a pedometer to quantify the exercise intensity and the relationship between the amount of exercise and carbohydrate metabolism in pregnant women with impaired

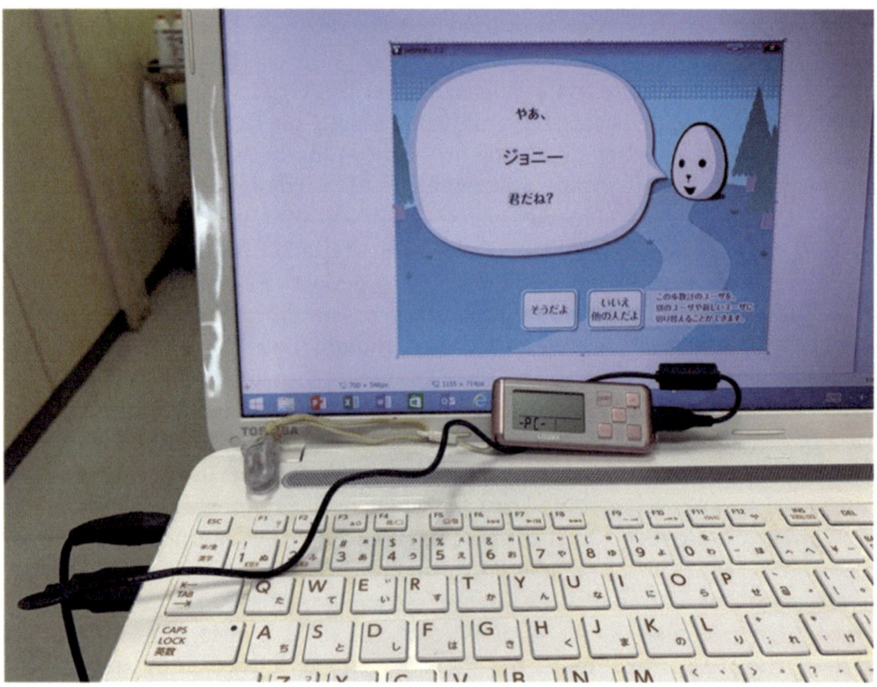

Figure 1.
Citizen digital pedometer TW700, connected to a laptop computer. The pedometer was connected to a laptop computer through a USB cable to upload steps.

DOI: http://dx.doi.org/10.5772/intechopen.93953

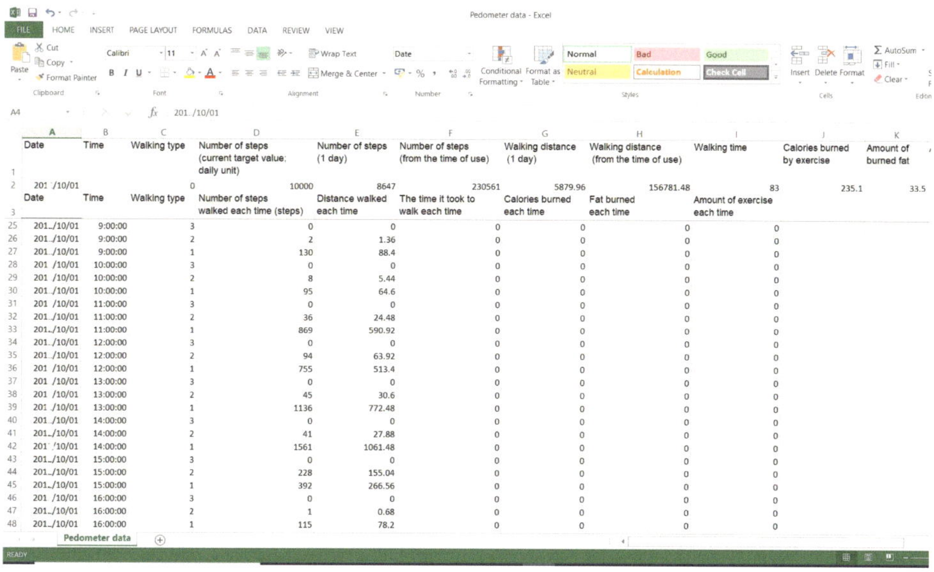

	A	B	C	D	E	F	G	H	I	J	K
1	Date	Time	Walking type	Number of steps (current target value: daily unit)	Number of steps (1 day)	Number of steps (from the time of use)	Walking distance (1 day)	Walking distance (from the time of use)	Walking time	Calories burned by exercise	Amount of burned fat
2	201 /10/01		0	10000	8647	230561	5879.96	156781.48	83	235.1	33.5
3	Date	Time	Walking type	Number of steps walked each time (steps)	Distance walked each time	The time it took to walk each time	Calories burned each time	Fat burned each time	Amount of exercise each time		
25	201 /10/01	9:00:00	3	0	0	0	0	0	0		
26	201 /10/01	9:00:00	2	2	1.36	0	0	0	0		
27	201 /10/01	9:00:00	1	130	88.4	0	0	0	0		
28	201 /10/01	10:00:00	3	0	0	0	0	0	0		
29	201 /10/01	10:00:00	2	8	5.44	0	0	0	0		
30	201 /10/01	10:00:00	1	95	64.6	0	0	0	0		
31	201 /10/01	11:00:00	3	0	0	0	0	0	0		
32	201 /10/01	11:00:00	2	36	24.48	0	0	0	0		
33	201 /10/01	11:00:00	1	869	590.92	0	0	0	0		
34	201 /10/01	12:00:00	3	0	0	0	0	0	0		
35	201 /10/01	12:00:00	2	94	63.92	0	0	0	0		
36	201 /10/01	12:00:00	1	755	513.4	0	0	0	0		
37	201 /10/01	13:00:00	3	0	0	0	0	0	0		
38	201 /10/01	13:00:00	2	45	30.6	0	0	0	0		
39	201 /10/01	13:00:00	1	1136	772.48	0	0	0	0		
40	201 /10/01	14:00:00	3	0	0	0	0	0	0		
41	201 /10/01	14:00:00	2	41	27.88	0	0	0	0		
42	201 /10/01	14:00:00	1	1561	1061.48	0	0	0	0		
43	201 /10/01	15:00:00	3	0	0	0	0	0	0		
44	201 /10/01	15:00:00	2	228	155.04	0	0	0	0		
45	201 /10/01	15:00:00	1	392	266.56	0	0	0	0		
46	201 /10/01	16:00:00	3	0	0	0	0	0	0		
47	201 /10/01	16:00:00	2	1	0.68	0	0	0	0		
48	201 /10/01	16:00:00	1	115	78.2	0	0	0	0		

Figure 2.
An example of the uploaded step data into a spreadsheet of Microsoft Excel.

		Correlation coefficient	P value
Relation between no. of steps and pre-prandial blood glucose level immediately following walking	No. of steps, morning & BL	−0.12	n.s.
	No. of steps, afternoon & BD	0.28	n.s.
	No. of steps, night & vds	0.25	n.s.
Relation between no. of steps and postprandial blood glucose level immediately following walking	No. of steps, morning & AB	0.06	n.s.
	No. of steps, afternoon & AL	0.02	n.s.
	No. of steps, night & AD	0.03	n.s.
Relation between total no. of steps per day and blood glucose level	Total no. of steps per day & vds	0.06	n.s.
	Total no. of steps per day & following day FBS	−0.02	n.s.
Relation between no. of steps per day and following day FBS	Insulin: yes	0.003	n.s.
	Insulin: no	−0.03	n.s.
Relation between no. of steps and change in blood glucose level before and after	No. of steps, morning & AB-BL	−0.12	n.s.
	No. of steps, afternoon & AL-BD	−0.24	n.s.
	No. of steps, night & AD-vds	−0.05	n.s.
	No. of steps, night & AD-following day FBS	−0.01	n.s.
	Total no. of steps per day & following day FBS-FBS	−0.08	n.s.

FBS: Pre-breakfast blood glucose, AB: After-breakfast blood glucose, BL: Pre-lunch blood glucose, AL: After-lunch blood glucose, BD: Pre-dinner blood glucose, AD: After-dinner blood glucose, vds: Bedtime blood glucose, n.s.: not significant.

Table 1.
Comparison of number of steps and blood glucose levels in 1-day based (from Ref. [34], with permission).

glucose tolerance employing a pedometer (Citizen Digital Pedometer TW 700 with high-sensitivity 3D acceleration sensor, CITIZEN SYSTEMS JAPAN CO., LTD, Japan) by which the recorded data of number of steps are stored chronologically for 30

		Correlation coefficient	P value
Relation of no. of steps per day and amount of change in HbA1c (comparison of 4-week based data)	**Entire pregnancy**	**−0.43**	**0.0263**
	Second trimester	**−0.64**	**0.0330**
	Third trimester	0.24	n.s.
Relation between avg. no. of steps and amount of change in GA (comparison of 4-week based data)	Entire pregnancy	−0.38	n.s. (0.082)
	Second trimester	−0.57	n.s. (0.109)
	Third trimester	0.24	n.s.
Relation between no. of steps per day and amount of change in maternal body weight (comparison of 2-week based data)	**Entire pregnancy**	**−0.49**	**0.0005**
	First trimester	−1(n = 2)	n.s.
	Second trimester	**−0.76**	**0.0003**
	Third trimester	−0.11	n.s.
Relation between no. of steps per day and average amount of insulin administered per day (comparison of 1-week based data)	**Entire pregnancy**	**−0.43**	**<0.0001**
	First trimester	0.69	n.s.
	Second trimester	**−0.42**	**0.0111**
	Third trimester	**−0.52**	**0.0005**
No. of steps per day for entire period and infant birthweight (SD score)		−0.22	n.s.

HbA1c: haemoglobin A1c, GA: Glycoalbumin, n.s.: not significant.

Table 2.
Comparison of average number of steps per day and all data items (from Ref. [34], with permission).

consecutive days [34]. The data stored in the pedometer are transferred through USB port of the computer and analysed chronologically (**Figures 1** and **2**). In a 24-hour time frame, there was no correlation between the number of steps walked and pre- or postprandial blood glucose level immediately after walking, nor between the average number of steps per day and the fasting blood glucose level on the next day (**Table 1**). However, the 4-week data showed that there was a negative correlation between the number of steps per day and the change in HbA1c levels (**Table 2**). Moreover, there was a negative correlation between the average number of steps per day and change in the maternal body weight (**Table 2**). A 1-week based data from the subjects administered with insulin indicated that there was a negative correlation between the average number of steps per day and the total amount of insulin administered per day. Our results indicated that pedometer-monitored walking improved insulin resistance without affecting blood glucose levels just after the bouts of walking. In addition, carrying the pedometer may have self-promoting effect for sustaining the exercise for the women with impaired glucose tolerance by noticing the improvement in the changes in the body weight and HbA1c levels in response to her steps walked. To conclude, our report was the first to show the usefulness of a pedometer for the management of IGT in pregnant women. We plan to continue studying this issue in future studies with higher numbers of participants along with nutritional counselling. Further studies are anticipated in order to design appropriate pedometer-monitored exercise plans not only for the management of IGT in pregnant women but also for that of the obese pregnant women. Nowadays, so many kinds of applications for pregnant women dealing with weight control, nutrition, foetal movement, maternal heart rates, it would be worthwhile to develop applications for incorporating pedometer data with body weight, maternal heart rate, ultrasound foetometric data and the parameters of the blood glucose control for the women with impaired glucose tolerance.

9. Conclusion

With the widespread use of smartphones equipped with pedometer function, walking exercises are easily monitored and utilised not only in normal but also in pregnant women with obesity and impaired glucose tolerance. Furthermore, data including footsteps, and pulse rates if smart watch will be used together with smartphone and information of the foetal growth, comprehensive management of the exercise and body weight control will be achieved. Further studies are expected to assess how many steps per day and how many bouts are optimal for the best blood sugar and body weight control during pregnancy.

Acknowledgements

We would like to thank Editage (www.editage.jp) for English language editing.

Conflict of interest

No conflict of interest exists.

Author details

Mariko Ueno[1], Mitsue Muraoka[2] and Koichiro Takagi[3]*

1 Department of Obstetrics and Gynecology, Tokyo Women's Medical University Medical Center East, Tokyo, Japan

2 Department of Obstetrics and Gynecology, Shiseikai Daini Hospital, Tokyo, Japan

3 Saigusa Maternity Clinic, Tokyo, Japan

*Address all correspondence to: kotak0821@gmail.com

References

[1] Hytten FE. Weight gain in pregnancy—30 year of research. S Afr Med J. 1981; 4(60):15-19.

[2] Karachaliou M, Georgiou V, Roumeliotaki T, Chalkiadaki G, Daraki V, Koinaki S, Dermitzaki E, Sarri K, Vassilaki M, Kogevinas M, Oken E, Chatzi L. Association of trimester-specific gestational weight gain with fetal growth, offspring obesity, and cardiometabolic traits in early childhood. Am J Obstet Gynecol 2015; 212:502.e1-14.

[3] Muraoka M, Takagi K, Ueno M, Morita Y, Nagano H. Fetal head growth during early to mid-gestation associated with weight gain in mothers with hyperemesis gravidarum: a retrospective Cohort study. Nutrients 2020;12, 1664;DOI:10.3390/nu12061664.

[4] LifeCycle Project-Maternal Obesity and Childhood Outcomes Study Group. Association of gestational weight gain with adverse maternal and infant outcomes. JAMA 2019;7:1702-1715.

[5] Institute of Medicine. Weight gain during pregnancy: reexamining the guidelines. Washington, DC: National Academies Press; 2009.

[6] Ministry of Health, Labour and Welfare (Guideline): Healthy Parents and Children 21: Diet and Lifestyle Guidance for Pregnant Women Investigation Committed, 2006 (in Japanese).

[7] Gesche J, Nilas L. Pregnancy outcome according to pre-pregnancy body mass index and gestational weight gain. Int J Obstet Gynecol Obstet 2015; 129:240-243.

[8] Yamori Y, Mochizuki M, Tojo N. Insulin and glucagon during pregnancy. Adv Obstet Gynecol. 1979;31:513-552.

[9] Kawanaka K. Exercise and skeletal muscle GLUT4. Trends in Academics. 2006;10:42-46 (in Japanese).

[10] Sanaka M. Diabetes and pregnant women. J Tokyo Women's Med Univ 2006; 76:389-393.

[11] ACOG Practice Bulletin No.190. Gestational diabetes mellitus. Obstet Gynecol. 2018;131(2):e49-e64.

[12] Diabetes Canada Clinical Practice Guidelines Epert Committee. 2018 Clinical Practice Guidelines Diabetes and Pregnancy. Can J Diabetes 2018;42:5255-5282.

[13] American College of Obstetricians and Gynecologists: Exercise during pregnancy and the postpartum period. Committee Opinion 2002, No. 267.

[14] Patel N, Godfrey KM, Pasupathy D, Levin J, Glynn AC Hayes L, B riley AL, Bell R, Lawlor DA, Oteng-Ntim E, Nelson SM, Robson SC, Sattar N, Singh C, Wardle J, White S, Seed PT, CStat, Poston L. Infant adiposity following a randomised controlled trial of a behavioural intervention in obese pregnancy. Int J Obes (Lond). 2017;41:1018-1026.

[15] Dempsey JC, Butler CL, Williams MA. No need for a pregnant women for a pregnant pause:Physical activity may reduce the occurrence of gestational diabetes mellitus and preeclampsia. Exerc Sport Sci Rev. 2005;33:141-149.

[16] Echeverria-Rodrigeuz O, Gallardo-Ortiz IA, Valle-Mondragon LD, Villalobous-Molina R. Angiotensin-(1-7) participates in enhanced skeletal muscle insulin sensitivity after bout of exercise.J Endocr Soc 2020;4:doi:1210/jendso/bvaa007.

[17] Artal R, Platt LD, Sperling M, Kammula RK, Jilel J, Nakamura R. Exercise in pregnancy. I. Maternal cardiovascular and metabolic responses in normal pregnancy. Am J Obstet Gynecol 1981;140:123-127.

[18] Soultanakis HN, Artal R, Wiswell RA. Prolonged exercise in pregnancy: glucose homeostasis, ventilatory and cardiovascular responses. Semin Perinatol. 1996;20(4):315-327. DOI: 10.1016/s0146-0005(96)80024-3

[19] Chapter 33: Role of exercise in reducing the risks of gestational diabetes mellitus in obese women. Raul Artal p.265-268. Lois G, Gian Carlo Di Renzo, Alberto De Leiva, Oded Langer. Textbook of Diabetes and Pregnancy (Maternal-fetal Medicine), Third edition. 2016.

[20] Plasqui G, Westerterp KR. Physical activity assessment with accelerometers: an evaluation against doubly labeled water. Obesity (Silver Spring). 2007;15(10):2371-2379. DOI: 10.1038/oby.2007.281

[21] Harrison CL, Thompson RG, Teede HJ, Lombard CB. Measuring physical activity during pregnancy. Int J Behav Nutr Phys Act. 2011;8:19. DOI: 10.1186/1479-5868-8-19

[22] Richardson CR, Newton TL, Abraham JJ, Sen A, Jimbo M, Swartz AM. A meta-analysis of pedometer-based walking interventions and weight loss. Ann Fam Med. 2008;6(1):69-77. DOI: 10.1370/afm.761

[23] Mitsui T, Shimaoka K, Tsuzuku S, Kajioka T, Sakakibara H. Pedometer-determined physical activity and indicators of health in Japanese adults. J Physiol Anthropol. 2008;27(4):179-184. DOI: 10.2114/jpa2.27.179

[24] Walker JR, Soroush A, Ainsworth BE, Belyea M, Swan PD, Yngve A. U.S. Cohort Differences in Body Composition Outcomes of a 6-Month Pedometer-Based Physical Activity Intervention: The ASUKI Step Study. Asian J Sports Med. 2014;5(4):e25748. DOI: 10.5812/asjsm.25748

[25] Nagelberg J, Burks H, Mucowski S, Shoupe D. The effect of home exercise on ovulation induction using clomiphene citrate in overweight underserved women with polycystic ovarian syndrome. Contraception and Reproductive Medicine 2016; 1:14 DOI 10.1186/s40834-016-0025-2.

[26] Huus K, Åkerman L, Raustorp A, Ludvigsson J. Physical Activity, Blood Glucose and C-Peptide in Healthy School-Children, a Longitudinal Study. PLoS One. 2016;11(6):e0156401. DOI: 10.1371/journal.pone.0156401

[27] Streuling I, Beyerlein A, Rosenfeld E, Hofmann H, Schulz T, von Kries R. Physical activity and gestational weight gain: a meta-analysis of intervention trials. BJOG. 2011;118(3):278-284. DOI: 10.1111/j.1471-0528.2010.02801.x

[28] Jiang H, Qian X, Li M, Lynn H, Fan Y, Jiang H, He F, He G. Can physical activity reduce excessive gestational weight gain? Findings from a Chinese urban pregnant women cohort study. International Journal of Behavioral Nutrition and Physical Activity.2012;9:12 http://www.ijbnpa.org/content/9/1/12.

[29] Cohen T, Koski KG. Limiting excess weight gain in healthy pregnant women: Importance of energy intakes, physical activity, and adherence to gestational weight gain guidelines. J of Pregnancy 2013;http://dx.doi.org/10.1155/2013/78032.

[30] Darvall JN, Wang A, Nazeem MN, et al. A Pedometer-Guided Physical

Activity Intervention for Obese Pregnant Women (the Fit MUM Study): Randomized Feasibility Study. JMIR Mhealth Uhealth. 2020;8(5):e15112. DOI: 10.2196/15112

[31] Mottola MF, Giroux I, Gratton R, et al. Nutrition and exercise prevent excess weight gain in overweight pregnant women. Med Sci Sports Exerc. 2010;42(2):265-272. DOI: 10.1249/MSS.0b013e3181b5419a

[32] Presset B, Laurenczy B, Malatesta D, Barral J. Accuracy of a smartphone pedometer application according to different speeds and mobile phone locations in a laboratory context. Journal of Exercise Science & Fitness. 2018; 16:43-48.

[33] Dahjio Y, Noubiap JJ, Azabji-Kenfack M, et al. Impact of a 12-week aerobic exercise training program on anthropometric and metabolic parameters of a group of type 2 diabetes Cameroonian women aged ≥50 years. Ann Transl Med. 2016;4(19):364. DOI: 10.21037/atm.2016.09.26

[34] Ueno M, Takagi K, Tachibana Y, et al. Quantitative analysis of exercise among pregnant women with impaired glucose tolerance using pedometer data: An observational study. J Obstet Gynaecol Res. 2020;46(3):396-404. DOI: 10.1111/jog.14164.